Metabolic Effects of Psychotropic Drugs

Modern Trends in Pharmacopsychiatry

Vol. 26

Series Editor

B.E. Leonard Galway

Metabolic Effects of Psychotropic Drugs

Volume Editors

J. Thakore Dublin
B.E. Leonard Galway

6 figures and 11 tables, 2009

KARGER

Basel · Freiburg · Paris · London · New York · Bangalore · Bangkok · Shanghai · Singapore · Tokyo · Sydney

Modern Trends in Pharmacopsychiatry
Formerly published as 'Modern Problems in Pharmacopsychiatry'

Dr. Jogin Thakore
Neuroscience Centre
St. Vincent's Hospital Fairview
Dublin (Ireland)

Prof. Brian E. Leonard
Department of Pharmacology
National University of Ireland
Galway (Ireland)

Library of Congress Cataloging-in-Publication Data

Metabolic effects of psychotropic drugs / volume editors, J. Thakore, B.E. Leonard.
p. ; cm. – (Modern trends in pharmacopsychiatry, ISSN 1662-2685 ; v. 26)
Includes bibliographical references and index.
ISBN 978-3-8055-9001-3 (hard cover : alk. paper)
1. Psychotropic drugs–Side effects. 2. Metabolic syndrome. 3. Schizophrenia–Chemotherapy–Complications. I. Thakore, Jogin H., 1962– II. Leonard, B. E. III. Series: Modern trends in pharmacopsychiatry ; v. 26.
[DNLM: 1. Psychotropic Drugs–adverse effects. 2. Psychotropic Drugs–metabolism. 3. Mental Disorders–drug therapy. W1 MO168P v.26 2009 / QV 77.2 M587 2009]
RM315.M456 2009
615'.788–dc22

Bibliographic Indices. This publication is listed in bibliographic services, including Current Contents® and Index Medicus.

www.karger.com
Printed in Switzerland on acid-free and non-aging paper (ISO 9706) by Reinhardt Druck, Basel
ISSN 1662-2685
ISBN 978–3–8055–9001–3

Contents

Preface

'There are no psychiatric patients, only medical patients with varying degrees of psychopathology.'

Schiffer RB, Klein RF, Sider RC: In: The Medical Evaluation of Psychiatric Patients. New York, Plenum, 1988, p. 28.

Patients suffering from major psychiatric disorders have reduced life expectancy. It is now well established that the increased morbidity and mortality is often caused by cardiovascular disease, cancer, inflammatory diseases and endocrine disorders such as type 2 diabetes. Yet it is only in recent years that attempts have been made to integrate the causes of physical illness with the underlying psychopathology of the disorder. Thus, it is now recognized that dysfunctional metabolism plays a crucial role in physical ill health that is associated with chronic psychiatric disorders such as depression and schizophrenia. Whether the metabolic syndrome is primarily caused by changes resulting from life style or the pathophysiology of the patient or, alternatively, is an important contribution to the psychopathology of the psychiatric disorder is an open question. A further complication relates to the impact of the drugs on the metabolism. Nowhere is this more apparent than in the reported effects of some atypical antipsychotics and antidepressants in causing weight gain, and possibly type 2 diabetes. Yet, as is apparent from several chapters in this volume it is uncertain whether the drugs cause the metabolic syndrome or that they exacerbate a vulnerability that exists in some major psychiatric disorders.

In this volume, the editors have brought together experts from clinical psychiatry, epidemiology, neuroimmunology, endocrinology and neuroscience to explore the different facets of the metabolic syndrome and its connection with the chronic effects of psychotropic drugs and with the psychopathology of some major psychiatric disorders.

Leonard puts forward the hypothesis that schizophrenia may be a low grade chronic inflammatory disorder by weaving together its possible viral, neurodevelopmental origins with recent evidence showing changes in various inflammtory markers such as IL-6 and TNF. Vemuri and coworkers focus on the important topic of insulin resistance and bipolar disorder with obesity, lifestyle choices and mood stabilizers playing important roles in women suffering from this mood disorder. Citrome and Vreeland discuss the topical and at times controversial issue of why obesity may develop in those mental illness and offer pertinent and practical solutions in the form of 'small steps' that may help the vast majority of patients to gain control over their weight and also discuss the possibility of using pharmacological and surgical interventions while Bushe focuses on the glucose abnormalities observed within chronic psychiatric disorders and the role of the illness versus antipsychotic agents. The author of this chapter poignantly observes that we still have not unraveled this complex relationship despite the explosion of information that we have witnessed over the last years. Based upon criteria set forth by the UK National Screening Committee, Holt and Peveler offer a compelling set of reasons for why type 2 diabetes and cardiovascular disease should be screened for in those with mental illness. Afzal and Thakore explore the relationship between stress, schizophrenia and the metabolic syndrome showing that a dysfunciotnal hypothalamic-pituitary-adrenal axis may be a common occurrence in both conditions and be partly responsible for their respective psychopathological and physical manifestations.

The chapter by Goethe and coworkers offers important metabolic insights into probably the most common psychiatric illness, namely depression. This chapter is a study which in effect details the rates of the metabolic syndrome in major depression and the various associations that may be related. In particular they find that atypical antipsychotics may not be associated with the higher than expected rates observed. Fitzgerald and Dinan then focus on how certain antipsychotics decrease dopaminergic activity leading to an increase in prolactin release which has potentially serious adverse effects ranging from lowering bone mineral density which can lead to fractures to being associated with breast and prostate cancer. Wildgust and Kohen discuss the propensity of antipsychotics to induce hyperprolactinemia which in turn can induce a lowering of bone mineral density, gynecomastia, galactorrhea and various menstrual cycle changes resulting in adverse hormonal profiles that could possibly potentiate the inherent risk that those with psychiatric illnesses have to cardiovascular disease.

This is the first monograph in a series devoted to pharmacopsychiatry. The aim of the series is to consider the inter-relationship between psychotropic drugs and the underlying psychopathology of psychiatric disorders. The current volume will consider the various aspects of the metabolic syndrome in major psychiatric disorders. Hopefully the contents of this first volume will be of interest not only to clinical psychiatrists but also to endocrinologists, immunologists, cardiologists and clinical neuroscientists.

Jogin Thakore
Brian E. Leonard

Thakore J, Leonard BE (eds): Metabolic Effects of Psychotropic Drugs.
Mod Trends Pharmacopsychiatry. Basel, Karger, 2009, vol 26, pp 1–11

Metabolic Syndrome and Schizophrenia: Is Inflammation the Cause?

Brian E. Leonard[a,b]

[a]Pharmacology Department, National University of Ireland, Galway, Ireland; [b]Department of Psychiatry and Psychotherapy, Ludwig Maximilians University, Munich, Germany

Abstract

Physical ill health is a common feature of schizophrenia. Hypertension, elevated cholesterol, obesity and type 2 diabetes are common occurrences and lead to increased morbidity and mortality. The question therefore arises whether these changes are due to an unhealthy life style of the patient or to a genetic predisposition that is exacerbated by life style and/or psychotropic medication. However, it is also possible that the metabolic changes that underlie physical ill health are a reflection of immune dysfunction. This review considers the evidence implicating an increase in inflammation in the psychopathology of schizophrenia, this being major contributory cause of diabetes and cardiovascular disease. It is concluded that there is substantial evidence to support this hypothesis and that more research is needed into the causal links between metabolic dysfunction and the psychopathology of schizophrenia in order to improve the physical, as well as the mental health, of the patient.

It is generally recognized that the ill health of the schizophrenic patient consists not only of psychiatric symptoms but also of physical illness. Thus, it has been estimated that the life expectancy for patients with schizophrenia is 20% lower that of the general population. Such premature death can result from increased risk of heart and cerebrovascular diseases while psychiatric co-morbidity includes alcohol and drug abuse which also contribute to the general ill health of the patient [1, 2].

Schizophrenia is associated with hypertension, obesity and elevated cholesterol [3]. Not surprisingly, the rates of the metabolic syndrome, type 2 diabetes and cardiovascular disease are higher than expected. The question therefore arises whether the increase in such conditions is a reflection of the patients unhealthy life style (lack of exercise and poor diet for example) or due to a genetic predisposition that is exacerbated by certain types of psychotropic medication. Furthermore, the increase in blood pressure, elevated cholesterol and diabetes are commonly associated with obesity in schizophrenic patients [3]. However, are these connections causal or co-incidental? If they are causally related, are they primarily due to the type of antipsychotic drug being administered to the patient and, if so, are some antipsychotics more likely to cause the metabolic syndrome than others? If the metabolic and physical changes are co-incidental then, presumably, by changing the life style of the patient such adverse changes should be reduced. These are some of the questions raised by the authors in this volume.

It is possible that the metabolic changes associated with schizophrenia are a reflection of immune dysfunction. Only in recent years has research established that there are clinically significant changes in the aspects of cellular and humoral immunity associated with the major symptoms of psychiatric disorders such as schizophrenia, bipolar disorder and depression [4, 5]. Furthermore, it is apparent that effective treatment of these disorders with psychotropic drugs largely attenuates the aberrant changes. The purpose of this chapter is to consider the possible involvement of inflammation as a common, possibly causal factor, in both the physical disorders and clinical symptoms that can accompany schizophrenia (fig. 1)

Immune Changes in Schizophrenia

The concept that a dysfunctional immune system plays a role in the etiology of schizophrenia can be traced back to the 19th century when it was estimated that approximately one-third of psychotic patients in Europe were suffering from neurosyphilis, a condition that has largely disappeared following the introduction of antibiotics in the 20th century. However, in the last century, it was observed that viral infections such as rubella and the influenza virus were also associated with the symptoms of schizophrenia, at least in some patients [6]. Perhaps the most compelling evidence for a link between schizophrenia and a dysfunctional immune system has been provided by Lindholm et al. [7] who demonstrated that a locus at chromosome 6p22 was linked to both schizophrenia and to the genes of the human lymphocyte (HLA) system. This system is crucially involved in combating viruses which might account for the increased vulnerability of schizophrenic patients to viral infections.

Another interesting connection between schizophrenia and the immune system has been provided by the susceptibility of first-degree relatives of schizophrenic patients to insulin-dependent diabetes mellitus. This susceptibility appears to be associated with the HLA locus on chromosome 6 [8]. Such an observation is particularly important because of the association between the metabolic syndrome and type 2 diabetes in schizophrenic patients being treated with the second-generation antipsychotic olanzapine. Clearly, there are differences in the genetic signal between type 1 and type 2 diabetes. Thus, there appears to be a decrease in the frequency of schizophrenia in patients with type 1 diabetes [9], which suggests that insulin, as such, is not directly linked to the pathology of schizophrenia. As is becoming apparent, type 2 diabetes is a possible consequence of dysfunctional metabolism initiated by immune, endocrine and mitochondrial changes that are symptomatic of schizophrenia.

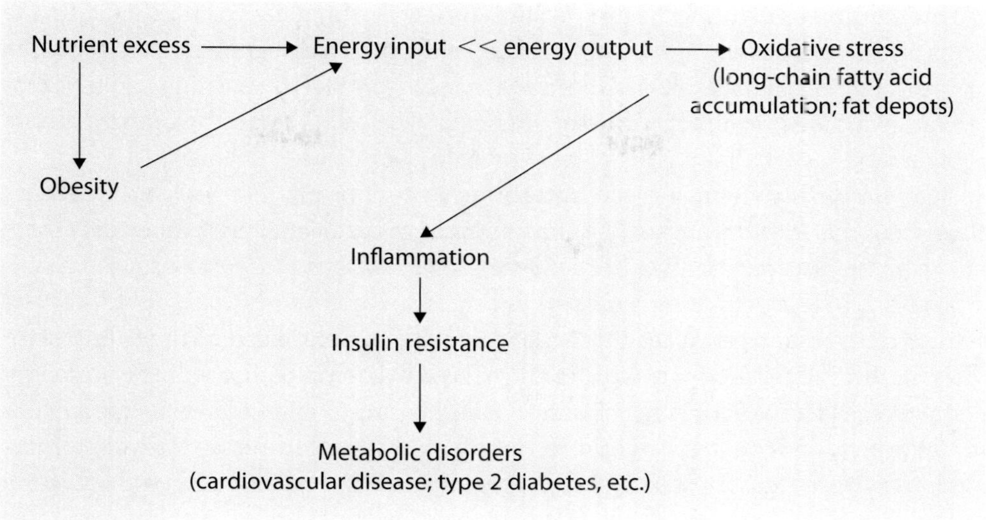

Fig. 1. Link between inflammation, obesity, diabetes and cardiovascular disease in schizophrenic patients.

Despite the circumstantial evidence linking viral infections to schizophrenia, no single virus has so far been identified as a causal agent. Furthermore, there is no evidence of a major immune reaction in the brains of schizophrenic patients; for example, no marked gliosis or evidence of lymphocyte infiltrates even though there is evidence of diffuse humoral reactivity in some patients. In addition, there is evidence that some of the peripheral immune changes are reflected in the brain [10, 11]. Leonard [10] has critically reviewed the evidence linking a disorder of the immune system to the psychopathology of schizophrenia

Evidence for the Activation of Cellular Immunity in Schizophrenia

In schizophrenia, there is evidence that the innate immune system is activated. Thus, the number of monocytes and some of the cytotoxic cells are increased [12]. In addition, the proportion of monocytes and macrophages in the CSF of patients with acute schizophrenia are increased, suggesting that immune activation occurs in the brain as well as in the periphery [13]. Of the pro-inflammatory cytokines that are raised in the CSF, interleukin 6 (IL-6) has been reported to be increased by a number of investigators [14]. IL-6 activates B cells, in addition to playing a key role in the inflammatory cytokine cascade, and therefore contributes to many of the immune changes seen in schizophrenia.

Il-6, in addition to other pro-inflammatory cytokines, is released from activated macrophages and monocytes in the periphery and from microglia and astrocytes in the brain. In vitro evidence has shown that IL-6 also stimulates the release of prolactin from the pituitary [15]. Whether this is relevant to the increase in the secretion of prolactin in patients being treated with antipsychotics is questionable as effective antipsychotic treatment usually attenuates the secretion of pro-inflammatory cytokines.

If IL-6 plays a role in the psychopathology of schizophrenia, to what extent do changes in this cytokine reflect the clinical status of the patient? It is clear that IL-6 is raised in the plasma of schizophrenic patients [15, 16] and that elevated plasma concentrations of this cytokine are related to both the duration of the disorder [17] and resistance to drug treatment [18]. In the CSF, the concentration of the soluble IL-6 receptor (sIL-6R) is also increased [18]. Il-6 has also been shown to activate both dopaminergic and serotonergic neurons in the hippocampus and the frontal cortex [19]. As these neurotransmitter changes have been implicated in the etiology of schizophrenia, it would appear that there is a close inter-relationship between the activation of the central and peripheral immune system and the changes in the monoamine neurotransmitters that are thought to be involved in the pathology of the disorder.

Although marked gliosis has seldom been detected in schizophrenic patients, microglial activation, triggered by the increase in the pro-inflammatory cytokines IL-1 and IL-6, has been detected in the frontal cortex [20]. It has also been observed that the expression of the IL-1 receptor antagonist (IL-1RA) is decreased in the prefrontal cortex of schizophrenic patients; this antagonist counteracts the overstimulation of IL-1 receptors by IL-1 [21]. As a consequence of the overactivation of IL-1, the hypothalamic-pituitary-adrenal axis is also activated; IL-1 is known to activate the anterior pituitary thereby enhancing the stress response [22]. IL-1 also decreases long-term potentiation in the hippocampus [23] thereby contributing to the disordered memory function frequently seen in patients with schizophrenia.

In addition to IL-6 and IL-1, other cytokines also appear to change in the plasma of schizophrenic patients. The changes in IL-2 and interferon-γ (IFN) were reported to be decreased, at least in some large-scale studies [24]. These findings suggest that there is a decrease in the Th-1 arm of the cellular immune system in patients with schizophrenia. It must be emphasized though that there are several conflicting findings in the literature regarding this conclusion [4, 25]. In the CSF, there is evidence that the IL-2 concentrations are increased in those patients who relapsed following treatment with haloperidol; these changes were associated with the recurrence of psychotic symptoms [24]. This may suggest that there is not a direct relationship between the blood and brain compartments of the immune system regarding the role of IL-2. On balance, it would appear that some schizophrenic patients show a shift in the adaptive immune system from cellular (Th1-mediated) to humoral (Th2-mediated) immunity. This shift appears to be more prominent in patients with predominantly negative symptoms that show a poor response to antipsychotic therapy [4, 25].

Schizophrenia is frequently considered to be a neurodevelopmental disorder that may arise as a consequence of prenatal exposure to a virus. Microglia are known to migrate into the brain early in development and to be involved in neural growth (low concentrations of pro-inflammatory cytokine have neuronal growth factor potential), pruning of neurons and removal of cell debris. Microglia therefore fulfil the role of macrophages in the brain and are involved in the presentation of antigens to phagocytic cells. They also release pro-inflammatory cytokines and are known to play a crucial role in immune function in schizophrenia so that an overactivation of the microglia contributes to the increased inflammatory challenge to the brain. Conversely, the astroglial cells have a largely neuroprotective role in the brain. There is evidence that the concentration of the S100 beta protein, derived from astroglial cells, is raised in patients independently of their medication [26], which has led to the suggestion that this change is in response to the neurodegenerative impact of the inflammatory mediators produced by the activated microglia.

Effect of Antipsychotic Drugs on the Immune Response in Schizophrenic Patients

Both in vitro and in vivo studies have suggested that effective antipsychotic treatment corrects the imbalance between the cellular and humoral arms of the adaptive immune system [4, 27]. Both haloperidol and clozapine, for example, have been shown to increase the release of IL-2 and IFN from whole blood cultures in vitro, whereas the antidepressant amitriptyline was ineffective [28]. In vivo, IL-18, a cytokine that also originates from activated Th-1 cells, is also increased following effective antipsychotic treatment, while the blunted reaction of patients to a salmonella vaccine challenge is reversed following effective drug treatment. In addition, the Th-3 cells have recently been implicated in correcting the imbalance between the Th-1 and Th-2 arms of the adaptive immune system. The Th-3 cells secrete transforming growth factors (TGF) of which serum TGF-1β has been reported to be elevated in schizophrenia [29]. This suggests that antipsychotic drug-induced changes in the concentration of TGF-1β might play a role in the normalization of the imbalance between the Th-1 and Th-2 arms of the immune system.

The activation of the B cells in schizophrenic patients to produce antibodies is an important part of humoral immunity and it would be anticipated that effective drug treatment would be correlated with an increase in antibody titer. There is ample clinical evidence that the antibody response to a vaccine challenge is reduced in schizophrenic patients but normalized on effective treatment [30]. Extensive studies have demonstrated that both the CD5 and B cells increase during long-term treatment with antipsychotic drugs [31]. Such findings lend further support to the view that there is an imbalance between the Th-1 and Th-2 systems which is corrected by effective antipsychotic treatment.

If inflammation plays a crucial role in the psychopathology of schizophrenia, then it would seem reasonable to postulate that anti-inflammatory drugs should have a therapeutic effect on the symptoms of the disorder. Prostaglandin E2 is a major inflammatory mediator in the brain and is synthesized by cyclo-oxygenase (COX) from arachidonic acid. Of the two COX enzymes in the brain, COX-2 is induced by pro-inflammatory cytokines. The product, prostaglandin 2, enhances the synthesis of Th-2 cytokines and inhibits the synthesis of Th-1 cytokines [32]. Of the COX-2 inhibitors that are available for clinical use in the treatment of arthritis, celecoxib is the most lipophilic. Recent clinical studies have demonstrated that in a prospective, double-blind, randomized trial of risperidone, alone or in combination with celecoxib, celecoxib significantly improved the positive and negative symptoms of the schizophrenic patients relative to those treated with risperidone alone [33]. This initial observation will hopefully lead to further studies of the use of anti-inflammatory agents in the treatment of schizophrenia.

On the Possible Role of Inflammation in Obesity and Type -2 Diabetes in Schizophrenia

It is well known that genetic and environmental factors interact to favor weight gain, changes which disrupt metabolism. The body fat stores are normally maintained within a narrow range by energy homeostasis. This process is controlled by the brain regions, such as hypothalamus, that control appetite and energy balance in addition to peripheral signaling systems that monitor energy stores. Glucose, free fatty acids, insulin and leptin are examples of the signaling molecules that activate the hypothalamus thereby controlling the metabolic rate and the desire to eat. Obesity does not simply arise from the passive accumulation of excess body weight but is an active adaptation to the elevation of body fat. Clearly, the genetic background of the individual contributes to the variation in the response to elevated body fat which helps to explain why some individuals are protected against weight gain while the majority is not despite the fact that they live in the same environment and eat the same food.

When energy intake exceeds expenditure, the resultant state of nutrient excess triggers responses in vascular endothelial cells, hepatocytes, myocytes, adipocytes, monocytes and macrophages resulting in metabolic dysfunction [34]. The cellular responses to the nutrient excess include the production of reactive oxygen species (ROS) that are generated by the mitochondrial oxidation of glucose and fatty acids. The resulting oxidative stress frequently results in cellular damage and triggers the inflammatory response [35]. Long-chain fatty acids and co-enzyme Q derivatives that are usually metabolized by the mitochondria also accumulate under these conditions and reflect a decrease in mitochondrial oxidative function. The final result of these changes is an activation of the C-jun N-terminal kinase and kappa-B pathways that promote inflammation. Thus inflammation appears to be a common end point of obesity.

The link between obesity and diabetes occurs as a result of a reduction in insulin function, thereby reducing the uptake of glucose into the target tissues. It is established that phosphotidylinositol-3-hydroxykinase, the inositol receptor substrate pathway, is particularly sensitive to inactivation by inflammatory mediators [36, 37]. Thus, with continuing nutrient excess tissues become insulin insensitive thereby leading to an extension of insulin resistance to most tissues as the inflammatory state progresses.

In addition to regulating nutrient utilization in peripheral tissues, the insulin receptor signaling system has been implicated in the actions of insulin and lepin on neuronal function. From experimental studies, it would appear that even short-term exposure to a palatable, energy-rich diet impairs the responsiveness of the hypothalamus to the effects of insulin and leptin [38]. This reduces the feedback regulatory mechanism whereby the brain normally reduces food intake in response to the increase in peripheral fat stores.

From the foregoing, it can be seen how inflammation participates in the link between obesity and type-2 diabetes. The 'beta-cell exhaustion hypothesis' of diabetes postulates that diabetes results when pancreatic beta cells fail to produce sufficient insulin due to insulin resistance thereby initiating type-2 diabetes [39].

Obesity is also linked to cardiovascular disease, both conditions occurring frequently in patients with schizophrenia. This is due to the impact of nutrient excess on the vascular endothelial cells. A major function of these cells is to activate nitric oxide synthase to produce the potent, but short-lived, vasodilator nitric oxide. The insulin receptor system-phosphoinositol-3-kinase pathway is a major factor in the control of nitric oxide synthesis in most tissues so that nutrient excess that reduces the activity of this pathway rapidly leads to a reduction in nitric oxide synthesis. Thus, the decrease in nitric oxide, combined with the accumulation of fat in the coronary circulation as a consequence of increased fat synthesis, provides a link between cardiovascular disease, diabetes obesity and inflammation [40].

While it is unlikely that the inhibition of the insulin-sensitive pathway by inflammatory mediators is the only factor of importance, it does emphasize the value of the integrative approach to studying metabolic disease and how such an approach may contribute to the physical ill health associated with major psychiatric disorders such as schizophrenia.

Role of Leptin in Inflammation and Its Possible Connection to Obesity in Schizophrenia

In most obese patients, obesity is associated with chronic low-grade inflammation of white adipose tissue. This results from the chronic activation of the innate immune system that subsequently leads to insulin resistance, impaired glucose tolerance and diabetes [41]. In obesity, the white adipose tissue is characterized by the increased synthesis and secretion of a range of inflammatory mediators such as tumor necrosis factor (TNF) and IL-6. In addition, the adipose tissue is infiltrated by macrophages that act as a major source of pro-inflammatory cytokines when activated. Conversely, weight loss leads to a reduction in the gene expression of the pro-inflammatory cytokines [42]. However, the adipocytes and macrophages are responsible for the increase not only of the pro-inflammatory cytokines but also for leptin and resistin. The increase in leptin exerts a strong negative feedback on insulin sensitivity thereby enhancing insulin resistance [43]. This situation is compounded by the impact of the glucocorticoids on the regulation of leptin; hypercortisolemia, a common feature of schizophrenia and other major psychiatric disorders, stimulates the release of leptin and thereby further enhances insulin resistance [44].

As has been mentioned previously, premature death due to cardiovascular disease is a common occurrence in both schizophrenia and depression. IL-6 is increased in both schizophrenia and major depression and is known to induce hepatic C-reactive protein that has been implicated in cardiovascular disease [45]. In addition to such changes, obesity is associated with a decrease in circulating adiponectin. Adiponectin is a cardioprotective agent that reduces the inflammatory action of pro-inflammatory cytokines such as TNF on the arterial walls and thereby protects against atherosclerosis [46].Thus a reduction in the availability of adiponectin in obesity indirectly contributes to an increase in vulnerability to cardiovascular disease. Figure 2 summarizes the link between impaired immunity, cardiovascular disease and obesity in schizophrenic patients.

Irrespective of the cause, epidemiological evidence suggests that obesity increases the risk of autoimmune disease and such immune related diseases as asthma. It has been speculated that this arises due to the decrease in immunological tolerance associated with the increase in the pro-inflammatory cytokines and leptin, and the decrease in adiponectin [47]. It has been demonstrated that both IL-6 and leptin downregulate the regulatory T cells thereby reducing antigen surveillance. Thus, obesity, through the induction of chronic low-grade inflammation and decreased immunological tolerance to antigens, increases the activity of the Th-2 humoral pathway thereby increasing the risk of allergies and immune-related disorders. Such changes are a common feature of schizophrenia.

Thus, in patients with schizophrenia a vicious cycle is created due to the inflammatory changes. These changes not only impact on the brain to contribute to the psychopathology of the disorder but are also responsible for the decline in physical health that characterizes such patients.

Conclusion

While physical ill health, commonly associated with schizophrenia, is frequently attributed to an unhealthy life style associated with lack of exercise, poor diet and smoking, it is now becoming apparent that there are underlying metabolic abnormalities that predispose patients to obesity and subsequent ill health. Superimposed on the metabolic abnormalities, antipsychotic drugs can contribute to the problem but it is presently unclear whether such drugs are the initiating cause of obesity, type

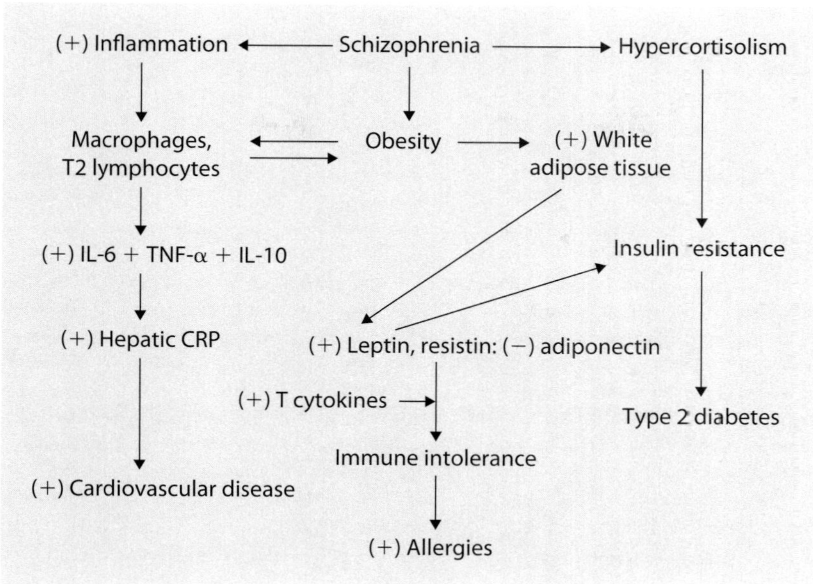

Fig. 2. Link between impaired immunity, obesity, diabetes and cardiovascular disease in patients with schizophrenia. (+) = Increase, (−) = decrease.

2 diabetes and heart disease. Clearly, there is now convincing evidence that there is an underlying disturbance of inflammatory pathways that initiates aberrant metabolic changes. While there is some evidence that effective treatment with antipsychotic drugs may attenuate such changes, it is clinically evident that a substantial proportion of patients still experience physical ill health. Whether the inflammatory changes are attenuated in such patients or not is unknown. Nevertheless, the results of such studies emphasize the need to expand research to investigate the broader aspects of metabolic function with a goal of developing treatments that are not only effective in ameliorating the psychiatric symptoms but also in improving the physical health of the patient.

References

1 Birkhofer A, Alger P, Schmid G, Foestl H: The cardiovascular risk of schizophrenic patients. Neuro psychiatry 2007;21:261–266.
2 Kozaric-Kovacic D, Folnegovic-Smak V, Folnegovic Z, Maruic A: Influence of alcoholism on the prognosis of schizophrenic patients. J Stud Alcohol 1995; 56:622–627.
3 Birkenaes AB, Birkeland KI, Engh JA, et al: Dyslipidaemia independent of body mass in antipsychotic treated patients under real life conditions. J Clin Psychopharmacol 2008;28:132–137.
4 Schwartz MJ, Mueller N, Riedel M, Ackenhail M: Markers of cellular and humoral immune activity: a shift in schizophrenia. Adv Biol Psychiatry 2001;20: 61–65.
5 Smith R: The macrophage theory of depression. Med Hypotheses 1991;35:298–306.
6 Moises HW, Ruger R, Reynolds GP, Fleckenstein B: Human cytomegalovirus DNA in the temporal cortex of a schizophrenic patient. Eur Arch Psychiatry Neurol Sci 1988;238:110–113.

7 Lindholm E, Elsholm R, Baleinniene J, et al: Linkage analysis of a large Swedish kindred provides further support for a susceptibility locus for schizophrenia on chromosome 6p23. Am J Med Genet 1999;88: 369–377.
8 Badenhoop K, Tonjes RR, Row H, et al: Endogenous retroviral long-terminal repeats of the HLA-DQ region are associated with susceptibility to insulin dependent diabetes mellitus. Hum Immunol 1996; 50:103–110.
9 Juvonen H, Reunanen A, Haukka J, et al: Incidence of schizophrenia in a nationwide cohort of patients with type 1 diabetes mellitus. Arch Gen Psychiatry 2007;64:894–899.
10 Mueller N, Ackenheil M: Psychoneuroimmunology, the cytokine network in the CNS and implication for psychiatric disorders. Prog Neuropsychopharmacol Biol Psychiatry 1998;22:1–31.
11 Leonard BE: Is there an immunological basis for schizophrenia? Expert Opin Clin Immunol 2005;1: 103–112.
12 Mueller N, Schlesinger BC, Hadjaniu M, et al: Cytotoxic T cells are elevated in unmedicated schizophrenic patients and related to blood-brain barrier and HLA allele DPA 02011. Schizophren Res 1998;12:69–71.
13 Nikkila HV, Muller K, Ahokas A, et al: Accumulation of macrophages in the CSF of schizophrenic patients during acute psychotic episodes. Am J Psychiatry 1999;156:1725–1729.
14 Maes M, Bosman E, CalabreseJ, et al: IL-2 and IL-6 in schizophrenia and mania: effects of neuroleptics and mood stabilisers. J Psychiatr Res 1995;29:141–152.
15 Spangelobl M, Judd AM, Isakson PC, MacLeod RM: IL-6 stimulates anterior pituitary hormone release in vitro. Endocrinology 1989;125:575–577.
16 Frommberger UH, Bauer J, Haselbauer P, et al: IL-6 plasma levels in depression and schizophrenia: comparison between the acute state and after remission. Eur Arch Psychiatr Clin Neurosci 1997;247: 228–232.
17 Ganguli R, Yang Z, Shurin G, et al: Serum IL-6 concentrations in schizophrenia: elevation associated with duration of illness. Psychiatr Res 1994;51:1–10.
18 Mueller N, Dobmeier P, Empel M, et al: Soluble IL-6 receptor in serum and CSF of paranoid schizophrenic patients. Eur Psychiatry 1997;12:294–299.
19 Zalcman S, Green-Johnson JM, Murray L, et al: Cytokine specific central monoamine alterations induced by IL-1,IL-2 and IL-6. Brain Res 1994;643: 40–49.
20 Radewicz K, Garey LS, Gentleman SM, Reynolds R: Increase in HLA-DR immunoreactive microglia in frontal and temporal cortex in chronic schizophrenics. J Neuropath Exp Neurol 2000;59:137–150.
21 Akiyama K: Serum levels of sIL-2R,IL-6 and IL-1RA in schizophrenics before and during neuroleptic administration. Schizophren Res 1999;37:97–106.
22 Sapolsky R, Rivier C, Yamamoto G, et al: IL-1 stimulates the secretion of hypothalamic CRF. Science 1987;238:522–524.
23 Vereker E, O'Donnell E, Lynch MA: The inhibitory effect of IL-1 beta on LTP is coupled with increased activity of stress activated protein kinase. J Neurosci 2000;20:6811–6819.
24 Arolt V, Rothermundt M, Wandinger KP, Kirchner H: Decrease in vitro production of interferon gamma and IL-2 in whole blood of patients with schizophrenia during treatment. Mol Psychiatry 2000;5:150–158.
25 Ganguli R, Brar JS, Chengappa KR, et al: Mitogen stimulated IL-2 production in never medicated first episode schizophrenics: the influence of age of onset and negative symptoms. Arch Gen Psychiatry 1995;52:878–882.
26 Rothermundt M, Ponath G, Glaser T, et al: S100 beta serum levels and long term improvement of negative symptoms in patients with schizophrenia. Neuropsychopharmacology 2004;29:1004–1011.
27 Cazzullo CL, Sacchetti E, Galluzzo A, et al: Cytokine profile in schizophrenic patients treated with risperidone: a three month follow-up study. Prog Neuropsychopharmacol Biol Psychiatry 2002;26:33–39.
28 Mueller N, Empel M, Riedel M, et al: Neuroleptic treatment increases sIL-2R and decreases IL-6R in schizophrenics. Eur Arch Psychiatr Clin Neurosci 1997;247:308–313.
29 Kim Y-K, Myint A-M, Lee B-H, et al: Th1,Th2 and Th3 cytokine alterations in schizophrenia. Neuropsychopharmacol Biol Psychiatry 2004;28: 1129–1134.
30 Ganguli R, Rabin BS, Kelly RH, et al: Clinical and laboratory evidence of autoimmunity in acute schizophrenia. Ann NY Acad Sci 1987;496:676–685.
31 Mueller N, Riedel M, Schwarz M, et al: Immunomodulatory effects of neuroleptics on the cytokine and cellular immune system in schizophrenia; in Wieselmann G (ed): Current Update in Psychoimmunology. Wien, Springer, 1992, pp 55–62.
32 Hinson RM, Williams JA, Shacter E: Elevated IL-6 induced by PGE2 in a murine model of inflammation: possible role of COX 2. Proc Natl Acad Sci USA 1996;93:4885–4890.
33 Mueller N, Riedel M, Scheppack E, et al: Beneficial antipsychotic effects of celecoxib add-on therapy compared to risperidone alone in schizophrenia. Am J Psychiatry 2002;159:1029–1034.
34 Wisse BE, Kim F, Schwartz MW: An integrative view of obesity. Science 2007;318:928–929.

35 De Souza CT, Araujo EP, Bordin S, et al: Consumption of a fat rich diet activates a proinflammatory response and induces insulin resistance in the hypothalamus. Endocrinology 2005;146:4192–4199
36 Hotamisligil GS: Inflammation and metabolic disorders. Nature 2006;444:860–867.
37 Lowell BB, Shulman GI: Mitochondrial dysfunction and type 2 diabetes. Science 2005;307:384–387.
38 Muenzberg H: Differential leptin access into the brain: a hierarchical organization of hypothalamic leptin target sites? Physiol Behav 2008;94:664–669.
39 Pan DA, Lillioja S, Kriketos AD, et al: Skeletal muscle triglyceride levels are inversely related to insulin action. Diabetes 1997;46:983–988.
40 Kim MJ, Maachi M, Debard C, et al: Increased adiponectin receptor-1 expression in adipose tissue of impaired glucose-tolerant obese subjects during weight loss. Eur J Endocrinol 2006;155:161–165.
41 Huypens P: Adipokines regulate systemic insulin sensitivity in accordance to existing energy reserves. Med Hypoth 2007;69:161–165.
42 Bastard JP: Leptin over expressed in adipocytes increases TNF alpha production and down regulates production of adiponectin. Eur Cytokine Netw 2006;17:4–12.
43 Dagogo-Jack S, Tykodi G, Umamaheswaran I: Inhibition of cortisol biosynthesis decreases circulating leptin levels in obese humans. J Clin Endocrinol Metab 2005;90:5333–5335.
44 Hersong LG, Linneberg A: The link between the epidemic of obesity and allergic diseases: does obesity induce decreased immune tolerance? Allergy 2007;62:1205–1213
45 Ladwig KH, Marten-Mittag B, Loewel H, et al: C-reactive protein, depressed mood, and the prediction of coronary heart disease in initially healthy men: results from the MONICA-KORA Augsburg Cohort Study. Eur Heart J 2005;26:2537–2542.
46 Osei K, Gaillard T, Schuster D: Plasma adiponectin levels in high-risk African-Americans with normal glucose tolerance, impaired glucose tolerance and type 2 diabetes. Obes Res 2005;13:179–185.

Brian E. Leonard, PhD, DSc
Department of Pharmacology
National University of Ireland
Galway (Ireland)
Tel. + 353 91 555 292, E-Mail belucg@iol.ie

Thakore J, Leonard BE (eds): Metabolic Effects of Psychotropic Drugs.
Mod Trends Pharmacopsychiatry. Basel, Karger, 2009, vol 26, pp 12–24

Insulin Resistance in Bipolar Women: Effects of Mood-Stabilizing Drugs

Mytilee Vemuri · Pascale Stemmle · Bowen Jiang · Anna Morenkova · Natalie Rasgon

Department of Psychiatry, Stanford University, Stanford, Calif., USA

Abstract

Women with bipolar disorder (BD) may have unique risk factors for insulin resistance (IR). Specific periods in a woman's reproductive timeline, specifically pregnancy and after the menopause, may represent times of increased IR. Moreover, women with BD demonstrate higher rates of obesity compared to men with BD, suggesting a sex-specific vulnerability to metabolic sequelae in BD. Additional contributors to metabolic sequelae, such as psychotropic medication, dysregulation of the hypothalamic-pituitary-adrenal axis, and genetic influences common in BD, may also manifest differently between the sexes. Several studies have suggested that women with BD may have more menstrual cycle irregularities than women in the general population. It has been hypothesized that such irregularities may be due to endocrinological disorders, such as polycystic ovarian syndrome or to hypothalamic-pituitary-adrenal axis dysfunction, both of which are also be associated with IR. Women treated with valproate may be particularly vulnerable to such irregularities. Lithium has not been observed to be associated with IR; however, it could theoretically influence IR through weight gain or effects of hypothyroidism. Treatment with atypical antipsychotics is associated with a greater risk of metabolic abnormalities, but sex-specific effects have not been observed. Definitive associations with IR have not thus far been demonstrated with either carbamazepine or lamotrigine.

High rates of metabolic disorders such as obesity, diabetes, lipid abnormalities and/or metabolic syndrome (MetS) have been observed in patients with bipolar disorder (BD). Insulin resistance (IR) often underlies metabolic disorders and has been hypothesized to be either (1) an underlying state predisposing both mood disorders and metabolic disorders; (2) a side effect of medications used to treat mood disorders, and/or (3) a consequence of mood disorders themselves (due to lifestyle changes or stress resulting from the disorder). Women with BD may represent a group needing specific treatment considerations. Sex differences in IR, unique metabolic sequelae of mood stabilizing medications in women, and reproductive events that may alter insulin-sensitivity are all factors that merit consideration in women with BD.

In 1988, Reaven [1] proposed that the cluster of IR (and by definition, hyperinsulinemia), impaired glucose tolerance, abnormalities of plasma lipids, and hypertension were part of a single syndrome, syndrome X. It has also been called the insulin resistance syndrome and, more commonly, the MetS. Insulin resistance is defined as a reduced responsiveness of a target cell or a whole organism to the insulin concentration to which it is exposed [2]. Thus, IR can lead to reduced cellular uptake of glucose, hyperglycemia, and resultant increased insulin production from the pancreas.

Sex Differences in Insulin Resistance

Insulin resistance can vary between sexes and across a women's reproductive life cycle. For example, some studies have suggested that girls through adolescence are inherently more insulin resistant than boys, but this relationship is thought to reverse after puberty [3, 4]. In adults, fat distribution patterns favor the development of IR in men, as men are more likely to develop abdominal obesity. Abdominal fat tissue is a major source of free fatty acids and cytokines and is associated with IR [5]. Premenopausal adult women more frequently develop peripheral obesity with subcutaneous fat accumulation, whereas men and postmenopausal women are more prone to central or abdominal obesity. After the menopause, concentrations of lipoproteins as well as body fat distribution shift to a more male pattern [5]. Pregnancy is also a time of elevated peripheral IR for women. During pregnancy, there is an approximate 50% reduction in insulin sensitivity by the third trimester; such changes are thought to be adaptive mechanisms to shunt nutrients to the developing fetus [6]. Glucose abnormalities can present differently between men and women. In a study of elderly people, the diagnosis of diabetes solely based on post-challenge hyperglycemia was more frequent in women than in men [7].

Individuals with Bipolar Disorder at Risk for Metabolic Disorders

The estimated prevalence of MetS or insulin resistance syndrome (IRS) in the USA is 24% in adults [8]. Many studies have demonstrated similarly high or higher rates of MetS in patients with BD, ranging from 16.7% to 49% [9–14]. Similarly, several retrospective studies have demonstrated an increased risk of diabetes in patients with BD [15–17]. Even patients without known diabetes or lipid abnormalities demonstrated high rates of diabetes (6.7%) and prediabetic glucose abnormalities (23.3%), including impaired fasting glucose and impaired glucose tolerance [10]. The majority of these BD patients were of normal weight, suggesting that metabolic abnormalities cannot entirely be explained by weight gain. Atypical antipsychotics such as olanzapine, risperidone and quetiapine are associated with the development or exacerbation of diabetes mellitus in bipolar patients [18]. However, one study has also shown medicated patients with BD are vulnerable to hyperinsulinemia, particularly those who gain weight or use beta-blockers, regardless of the type of psychotropic used [18a]. We reported high rates of IR in all of our studies in women with BD, regardless of the type of psychotropic medication used [19–22]. Metabolic dysfunction may also be present *prior* to psychotropic treatment – recent data from our group [22a] found high rates of metabolic dysfunction and obesity in a small sample of untreated women with BD. Therefore, additional factors such as concurrent therapy with other drugs, genetic influences, and the pathophysiological etiology of the BD illness itself may contribute to IR.

Intrinsic neuroendocrine features of BD may lead to somatic metabolic dysfunction. In both the depressive and manic phases of BD, there is a positive association with chronic stress and elevated cortisol [23]. These abnormalities, along with frequent hyperactivity of the hypothalamic-pituitary-adrenal (HPA) axis, could potentially contribute to the higher prevalence of MetS. Chronically elevated glucocorticoids from HPA hyperactivation impedes glucose uptake by insulin, which in turn promotes metabolic dysfunction and cardiovascular disease [24]. Dysregulation of the HPA axis is also associated with obesity and elevated levels of leptin, a hormone that mediates central regulation of body mass, suggesting that the obesity may be due to inefficient leptin signaling and decreased feelings of satiety [23]. Another consequence of elevated cortisol is increased activity of lipoprotein lipase, which increases the amount of adipose tissue [25]. Elevated cortisol secretion also causes IR in muscles and affects the function of glycogen synthase, which can then promote peripheral IR [26, 27].

Specific Metabolic Features of Women with Bipolar Disorder

Metabolic Syndrome

Baseline data from the Clinical Antipsychotic Trial of Intervention Effectiveness (CATIE) demonstrated higher rates of MetS in women with schizophrenia (51.6%), when compared with women in the general population and with men with schizophrenia (36.0%) [18]. However, gender differences in MetS prevalence in BD patients have not emerged as clearly. The majority of studies of prevalence rates of MetS in BD have not noted significant gender differences, but have involved smaller numbers than those in the CATIE study [12, 13]. One study demonstrated a higher prevalence of MetS in bipolar women in comparison with bipolar men [14].

Obesity

Individuals with BD demonstrate higher rates of obesity than the general population [28]. Women with BD appear to have higher rates of obesity than men with BD [29], and a propensity towards higher waist circumferences [10]. Obese patients with either BD or schizophrenia are more likely to be women [30], and weight gain has been shown to be associated with female sex [31]. An evaluation of data from the Systematic Treatment Enhancement Program for Bipolar Disorder (STEP-BD) demonstrated greater rates of obesity in bipolar women (31%), compared to bipolar men (21%); in contrast, there were greater rates of overweight in bipolar men (38%), compared to women (22%) [32], a finding consistent with previous studies [33]. Women with BD appear to have a higher likelihood of increased waist circumference than men with BD, suggesting a sex-specific vulnerability to IR in BD. Changes in weight and appetite are found more commonly in women than in men with BD [34, 35]. Higher rates of thyroid and eating disorders are seen in women with BD [36]. Factors that influence the onset and maintenance of obesity in BD include both gender and eating behavior [37]. Similarly, both sex and eating disorders significantly correlate with overweight and obesity in BD [33]. Sex differences in comorbid thyroid disease, bulimia, and appetite changes could theoretically lead to more weight gain in bipolar women.

Menstrual Irregularities and Bipolar Disorder

Several studies have suggested that women with BD may have more menstrual cycle irregularities than women in the general population. It has been hypothesized that such irregularities are due to endocrinological disorders, specifically polycystic ovarian syndrome (PCOS) or due to HPA dysfunction, both of which could be associated with IR and metabolic dysfunction.

PCOS is one of the most common endocrine disorders occurring in reproductive-aged endocrine disorder with an estimated prevalence of between 4 and 6% [38]. It is characterized by chronic anovulation and hyperandrogenism [39]. Chronic anovulation can lead to menstrual abnormalities and infertility. Hyperandrogenism can manifest as hirsutism (excess hair growth on the face), acne, and male-pattern balding. Metabolic consequences of PCOS include obesity and IR which may lead to type-2 diabetes mellitus and cardiovascular disease (CVD) [39–42], and underscores the relationship between reproductive abnormalities and IR in women. PCOS is associated with overweight or obesity in approximately 50% of women with the disorder [43]. Even if they are normal weight, individuals with PCOS tend to have a higher proportion of abdominal body fat [44, 45], which is a risk factor for both IR [46] and CVD [47]. Lipid abnormalities have also been found at high rates among women with PCOS, including low high-density lipoprotein cholesterol (HDL-C) levels and elevated triglyceride levels [48, 49]. Women with PCOS may also exhibit increased immunological responses, such as elevated high sensitivity C-reactive protein (hsCRP) and interleukin-6 (IL-6), which can lead to subclinical CVD and impairment of endothelial structure [50–53]. Thus, the development of PCOS may present significant medical complications for many women.

Mood Stabilizers and Impact on Insulin Resistance in Women with Bipolar Disorder

Women with BD are often treated with psychotropic agents, including mood stabilizers, atypical antipsychotics, and antidepressants, whose effects on reproductive function and IR are not fully understood. Medications may impact weight and endocrine abnormalities in a variety of ways that contribute to IR. For example, it has been theorized that valproate can influence the development of menstrual abnormalities by decreasing estrogen levels, increasing luteinizing hormone and increasing testosterone [54]. The increase in testosterone can lead to an arrest in maturation of ovarian follicles, leading to the development of polycystic ovaries. Additionally, valproate may cause an increase in leptin resulting in increased body weight [54], or lead to glucose-stimulated insulin secretion by pancreatic cells [55]. Weight gain itself, not specific to valproate use, may lead to menstrual abnormalities or IR. In our studies, we demonstrated a correlation between BMI and both testosterone and insulin levels in women with BD [54]. Weight gain on psychotropic medications also predicted new onset menstrual abnormalities [54]. Thus, weight gain (whether it is inherent to BD or a result of any weight-liable mood stabilizer) may contribute to IR, particularly in women.

Here, we review the evidence for the association between certain medications implicated in IR.

Valproate

Valproate has been reported to have associations with PCOS in women with epilepsy and BD. Concerns over an association between valproate and PCOS first arose in valproate-treated women with epilepsy who were found to have high rates of PCOS [56]. As valproate is commonly used to treat women with BD, questions about its possible impact on endocrine and reproductive function in psychiatric populations emerged. Several cross-sectional studies have found increased rates of PCOS, menstrual abnormalities and/or hyperandrogenism in bipolar patients using valproate [22, 57, 58]. A study of 38 bipolar women [58] receiving either valproate or lithium monotherapy for at least 2 years demonstrated higher rates of menstrual abnormalities in patients receiving valproate (50%) than in patients receiving lithium (15%). Menstrual abnormalities were more prevalent in overweight/obese patients than in lean patients. Free testosterone and androstenedione levels were significantly higher than the reference range in valproate-treated patients, and luteinizing hormone was elevated in both groups. A similar study demonstrated that women receiving valproate had a significantly greater rate of menstrual abnormalities (47%) than women receiving non-valproate therapy (13%) and control women (0%) [57]. Forty-one percent of women with BD taking valproate had PCOS. A larger study of 300 women in the STEP-BD study found 10.6% (n = 9) of 86 patients treated with valproate had new onset menstrual cycle irregularities and hyperandrogenism within the first year of valproate use, most of of whom were also obese and had IR [59]. A follow-up study demonstrated reversal of PCOS reproductive features in 3 of 4 women upon discontinuation of valproate, while symptoms continued in 3 women continuing valproate [60].

Our own findings on this topic have yielded mixed results about the association of valproate with PCOS features; however we have consistently shown high rates of menstrual abnormalities in women with BD, even preceding diagnosis and treatment for the disorder. A pilot study of 22 women with BD, receiving lithium monotherapy, valproate monotherapy, or lithium-valproate combination therapy did not reveal a significant association between PCOS and valproate or lithium therapy [19]. All patients on lithium monotherapy or combination therapy and 60% of patients on valproate monotherapy reported menstrual disturbances. There were no significant differences in BMI or hirsutism, and hormone levels were within normal limits for all 3 groups. None of the subjects met NIH-defined criteria for PCOS. In a follow-up cross-sectional study [22], we examined 80 reproductive-aged women who were receiving valproate therapy or non-valproate therapy for BD. Fifty-two of the 80 women (65%) reported current menstrual abnormalities, 40 of which (50%) reported one or more menstrual abnormalities that preceded the diagnosis of BD. Fifteen women (38%) reported developing menstrual abnormalities since beginning treatment for BD, 14 of whom developed abnormalities since treatment with valproate. No significant differences were observed between valproate and non-valproate groups in mean levels of free or total serum testosterone. Three of the 50 women (6%) taking valproate met the criteria for PCOS, compared to 0% of the 22 taking other mood-stabilizer medications.

We conducted the first longitudinal study of this relationship, evaluating reproductive endocrine and metabolic markers in 25 women treated for BD over a 2-year time period [21]. At baseline, 10 (40%) women were currently undergoing treatment with valproate. Consistent with other published reports described above, 41.7% of subjects reported current oligomenorrhea, while 40% reported oligomenorrhea before starting medication. Rates of oligomenorrhea and clinical hyperandrogenism did not differ by type of medication use. Eighty percent of all subjects had a high homeostatic model assessment of IR (HOMA-IR) at baseline. Valproate use was associated with an increase over time in total testosterone. In contrast to other studies, we did not find co-occurrence of new-onset menstrual abnormalities with hyperandrogenism. We concluded that oligomenorrhea, hyperandrogenism, and IR are common in women with BD, and increases in androgen hormones may be related to valproate use [21].

Lithium

Lithium could theoretically influence IR in women through weight gain or through effects of hypothyroidism. Lithium exposure increases the incidence of hypothyroidism. Clinical and subclinical hypothyroidism is more commonly seen in women than men with BD and in the general population, and the risk increases with age [61–63]. Hypothyroidism can cause alterations in lipid metabolism, weight gain, and menstrual cycle abnormalities, which in turn could impact IR.

Lithium treatment in patients with BD has been associated with weight gain in numerous studies [64–68] and has been found to range from 5 kg within 1–2 years to 4.5–15.6 kg over 2 years [69, 70]. A recent animal study found that lithium increased gastrointestinal weight of male and female rats but only increased total body weight in females [71]. The mechanisms for lithium-induced weight gain remain unclear despite several conjectures. Lithium appears to exert insulin-like activity on carbohydrate metabolism, leading to increased glucose absorption in adipose tissue [72–75]. Lithium may also have direct effects on the hypothalamus to stimulate appetite and/or thirst and can also result in increased fluid retention [76]. Although lithium treatment can result in significant weight gain and/or hypothyroidism, long-term lithium treatment does not appear to be associated with IR or increased risk of developing diabetes mellitus [66]. In fact, one study suggested that lithium exerts anti-diabetic effects by lowering blood glucose levels in a manic-depressive female with adult onset diabetes mellitus [77].

Atypical Antipsychotics

Atypical antipsychotic (AAP) treatment is also associated with a greater risk of metabolic abnormalities, such as dyslipidemia, weight gain, and new-onset type 2 diabetes mellitus [78]. Sex-specific impacts of atypical antipsychotics on IR have not been elucidated. Recent data suggest that AAPs may be more weight-liable medications than valproate [79]. In general, clozapine and olanzapine treatment are associated with the greatest risk of weight gain, while risperidone, quetiapine, ziprasidone, aripiprazole, amisulpride and zotepine have relatively lower levels of risk [80, 81]. In several studies examining IR via glucose tolerance testing, patients who received clozapine or olanzapine demonstrated higher degrees of resistance compared with those treated with risperidone [82–84]. Furthermore, in a recent study of 242 patients, patients treated with olanzapine or clozapine had significantly higher prevalence of dyslipidemia compared to unmedicated patients, independent of BMI [85]. A large matched case-control study of patients treated with AAPs conducted by Olfson et al. [86] found that treatment with clozapine, risperidone, quetiapine, olanzapine, ziprasidone, but not aripiprazole, was associated with a significant risk for hyperlipidemia, as compared to no AAP medication.

There is clear correlation between obesity and IR, as adipocytes secrete several hormones (leptin, adipsin, adiponectin, tumor necrosis factor-α) that impair insulin secretion and/or insulin effects [87]. With the exception of adiponectin, all the hormones secreted by the endocrine adipose tissue exert antagonistic effects on insulin secretion and action [88]. As mentioned above, the use of AAPs is strongly associated with clinical weight gain and obesity; therefore, IR may be the result of increased adipose tissue and their hormone secretions. AAPs can also produce hyperinsulinemia through their antagonistic effects on dopamine (D2) receptors. D2 receptors are expressed in the β-cells and mediate glucose-stimulated secretion of insulin. Impaired dopamine receptor activation by via the effects of AAP may result in a compensatory increase in insulin secretion, which over time may develop into insulin insensitivity and resistance [89, 90]. Hormones important to appetite regulation and maintenance of adipose homeostasis such as leptin (anorectic) and ghrelin (orexigenic) may be disrupted by AAP treatment. It is hypothesized that AAP treatment disrupts appetite regulation by increasing ghrelin and/or decreasing leptin, thereby increasing Agouti-related peptide (AGRP), neuropeptide Y (NP-Y), and orexin, leading to increased food intake and obesity. Ghrelin levels in patients treated with AAP for 1 year were significantly higher than in placebo-treated controls, with no difference between the various atypical agents that were used (clozapine, olanzapine, risperidone, or quetiapine) [91]. However, several other reports have indicated no difference in ghrelin levels or a reduction in ghrelin levels [92–94].

Carbamazepine, Lamotrigine

Carbamazepine (CBZ) may be associated with weight gain and metabolic abnormalities, but to a lesser extent than valproate or lithium [95]. In a study of 105 epileptic women treated with valproate and CBZ monotherapy, rates of PCOs were similar (in both groups) to rates in the general population. However, BMI, triglycerides, and postprandial insulin were higher in valproate-treated patients than CBZ-treated patients. Of note, the enzyme-inducing properties of CBZ may reduce levels of free and total thyroxin in patients with thyroid dysfunction [96]. To date, the literature has not supported an association between lamotrigine (LTG) and IR. In a study of 54 women with epilepsy, MetS was more frequently associated with VPA-treated patients (41.7%) than CBZ (5.3%), LTG (0%), or topiramate (TPM) groups (0%) [97]. A post-hoc analysis was performed from a 12-week prospective open-label study of 1,175 patients with BD initiated on lamotrigine either as monotherapy or adjuvant treatment to valproate, lithium, antipsychotics, or antidepressants. No weight or BMI changes were noted after lamotrigine monotherapy or adjuvant therapy [98]. These findings are consistent with studies of lamotrigine in epilepsy populations [99].

Topiramate and Zonisamide

While not approved for use as mood stabilizers, topiramate and zonisamide have potential roles in treating patients with BD. Both medications are considered weight neutral, and may possibly even contribute to weight loss. In patients with epilepsy and type 2 diabetes, patients showed better glycemic control when treated with topiramate [100]. Evidence has supported the utility of topiramate in treating binge-eating episodes in patients with obesity [101]. Both topiramate and zonisamide may have a role in promoting weight loss in patients with BD [102].

Conclusions

A growing literature supports an association between insulin resistance and bipolar disorder in women. Obesity in itself is a major contributor to IR and is a is highly prevalent in BD, more so in women with BD.

Women with BD may be at risk for insulin resistance even prior to mood stabilizer initiation, and may also be susceptible to additional risks with certain mood stabilizers as weight gain associated with intake of these agents may further increase risk of insulin resistance. Mood stabilizing drugs confer variable metabolic risks. Valproate in particular has been implicated in development of IR as a component of PCOS. Valproate, lithium, and CBZ may cause weight gain, which can cause or worsen insulin resistance. Hypothyroidism, a side effect of lithium, may also be associated with weight gain and again is more prominent in women with BD than men. Many of the second-generation antipsychotics, including olanzapine, risperidone, and quetiapine, have been implicated in weight gain, and glucose and lipid abnormalities independent of weight gain.

Mood stabilizers likely play only a partial role in the development of insulin resistance and metabolic disorders in women with BD, and likely interact with a number of other features including patient genetics, baseline weight, and psychiatric illness. Therefore, inquiry into an individual patient's medical and family history, particularly diabetes, hyperlipidemia, hypertension, obesity, and metabolic side effects of previous medication, is a critical part of medication management. Longitudinal, prospective studies needed to further describe the interaction between mood disorders, insulin resistance and mood stabilizing drugs used in its treatment. Further research needs to delineate gender differences in the effects of medications used to treat psychiatric disorders, and ultimately to develop specialized treatment strategies for women with bipolar disorder. In the meantime, clinicians are charged with the task of reducing the medical burden of insulin resistance and metabolic disorders in patients with major mental illnesses.

References

1 Reaven GM: Banting lecture 1988: role of insulin resistance in human disease. Diabetes 1988;37:1595–1607.

2 Shanik MH, Xu Y, Skrha J, Dankner R, Zick Y, Roth J: Insulin resistance and hyperinsulinemia: is hyperinsulinemia the cart or the horse? Diabetes Care 2008;31(suppl 2):S262–S268.

3 Moran A, Jacobs DRJ, Steinberger J, et al: Changes in insulin resistance and cardiovascular risk during adolescence: establishment of differential risk in males and females. Circulation 2008;117:2361–2368.

4 Travers SH, Jeffers BW, Bloch CA, Hill JO, Eckel RH: Gender and Tanner stage differences in body composition and insulin sensitivity in early pubertal children. J Clin Endocrinol Metab 1995;80:172–178.
5 Regitz-Zagrosek V, Lehmkuhl E, Weickert MO: Gender differences in the metabolic syndrome and their role for cardiovascular disease. Clin Res Cardiol 2006;95:136–147.
6 Galerneau F, Inzucchi SE: Diabetes mellitus in pregnancy. Obstet Gynecol Clin North Am 2004;31:907–933, xi-xii.
7 Barrett-Connor E, Ferrara A: Isolated postchallenge hyperglycemia and the risk of fatal cardiovascular disease in older women and men. The Rancho Bernardo Study. Diabetes Care 1998;21:1236–1239.
8 Ford ES, Giles WH, Dietz WH: Prevalence of the metabolic syndrome among US adults: findings from the third National Health and Nutrition Examination Survey. JAMA 2002;287:356–359.
9 Yumru M, Savas HA, Kurt E, et al: Atypical antipsychotics related metabolic syndrome in bipolar patients. J Affect Disord 2007;98:247–252.
10 Van Winkel RDHM, Hanssens L, Wampers M, Scheen A, Peuskens J: Prevalence of diabetes and the metabolic syndrome in a sample of patients with bipolar disorder. Bipolar Disorders 2008;10:342–348.
11 Fagiolini A, Frank E, Scott JA, Turkin S, Kupfer DJ: Metabolic syndrome in bipolar disorder: findings from the Bipolar Disorder Center for Pennsylvanians. Bipolar Disord 2005;7:424–430.
12 Cardenas J, Frye MA, Marusak SL, et al: Modal subcomponents of metabolic syndrome in patients with bipolar disorder. J Affect Disord 2008;106:91–97.
13 Garcia-Portilla MP, Saiz PA, Benabarre A, et al: The prevalence of metabolic syndrome in patients with bipolar disorder. J Affect Disord 2008;106:197–201.
14 Teixeira PJ, Rocha FL: The prevalence of metabolic syndrome among psychiatric inpatients in Brazil. Rev Bras Psiquiatr 2007;29:330–336.
15 Lilliker SL: Prevalence of diabetes in a manic-depressive population. Compr Psychiatry 1980;21: 270–275
16 Cassidy F, Ahearn E, Carroll BJ: Elevated frequency of diabetes mellitus in hospitalized manic-depressive patients. Am J Psychiatry 1999;156:1417–1420.
17 Regenold WT, Thapar RK, Marano C, Gavirneni S, Kondapavuluru PV: Increased prevalence of type 2 diabetes mellitus among psychiatric inpatients with bipolar I affective and schizoaffective disorders independent of psychotropic drug use. J Affect Disord 2002;70:19–26.
18 Guo JJ, Keck PE Jr, Corey-Lisle PK, et al: Risk of diabetes mellitus associated with atypical antipsychotic use among Medicaid patients with bipolar disorder: a nested case-control study. Pharmacotherapy 2007; 27:27–35.
18a Tsai SY, Lee HC, Chen CC: Hyperinsulinaemia associated with beta-adrenoceptor antagonist in medicated bipolar patients during manic episode. Prog Neuropsychopharmacol Biol Psychiatry 2007; 31(5);1038–1043.
19 Rasgon NL, Altshuler LL, Gudeman D, et al: Medication status and polycystic ovary syndrome in women with bipolar disorder: a preliminary report. J Clin Psychiatry 2000;61:173–178.
20 Rasgon N, Bauer M, Glenn T, Elman S, Whybrow PC: Menstrual cycle related mood changes in women with bipolar disorder. Bipolar Disord 2003; 5:48–52.
21 Rasgon NL, Reynolds MF, Elman S, et al: Longitudinal evaluation of reproductive function in women treated for bipolar disorder. J Affect Disord 2005;89:217–225.
22 Rasgon NL, Altshuler LL, Fairbanks L, et al: Reproductive function and risk for PCOS in women treated for bipolar disorder. Bipolar Disord 2005;7:246–259.
22a Stemmle PG, Kenna HA, Wang PW, Hill SJ, Ketter TA, Rasgon NL: Insulin resistance and hyperlipidemia in women with bipolar disorder. J Psychiatr Res 2008, May 17.
23 Cassidy F, Ritchie J, Carroll B: Plasma dexamethasone concentration and cortisol response during manic episodes. Biol Psychiatry 1998;43:747–754.
24 Brindley D, Rolland Y: Possible connections between stress, diabetes, obesity, hypertension and altered lipoprotein metabolism that may result in atherosclerosis. Clin Sci (Lond) 1989;77:453–461.
25 Bjorntorp P: The regulation of adipose tissue distribution in humans. Int J Obes Relat Metab Disord 1996;20:291–302.
26 DeFronzo R, Ferrannini E: Insulin resistance: a multifaceted syndrome responsible for NIDDM, obesity, hypertension, dyslipidemia, and atherosclerotic cardiovascular disease. Diabetes 1991;14:173–194.
27 Bowden CL, Calabrese JR, McElroy SL, et al: A randomized, placebo-controlled 12-month trial of divalproex and lithium in treatment of outpatients with bipolar I disorder Divalproex Maintenance Study Group. Arch Gen Psychiatry 2000;57:481–489.
28 Elmslie JL, Silverstone JT, Mann JI, Williams SM, Romans SE: Prevalence of overweight and obesity in bipolar patients. J Clin Psychiatry 2000;61:179–184.
29 Arnold LM: Gender differences in bipolar disorder. Psychiatr Clin North Am 2003;26:595–620.
30 Kolotkin RL, Corey-Lisle PK, Crosby RD, et al: Impact of obesity on health-related quality of life in schizophrenia and bipolar disorder. Obesity (Silver Spring) 2008;16:749–754.
31 Taylor V, MacQueen G: Associations between bipolar disorder and metabolic syndrome: a review. J Clin Psychiatry 2006;67:1034–1041.

32 Wang PW, Sachs GS, Zarate CA, et al: Overweight and obesity in bipolar disorders. J Psychiatr Res 2006;40:762–764.
33 McElroy SL, Frye MA, Suppes T, et al: Correlates of overweight and obesity in 644 patients with bipolar disorder. J Clin Psychiatry 2002;63:207–213.
34 Kawa I, Carter JD, Joyce PR, et al: Gender differences in bipolar disorder: age of onset, course, comorbidity, and symptom presentation. Bipolar Disord 2005;7:119–125.
35 Benazzi F: Gender differences in bipolar II and unipolar depressed outpatients: a 557-case study. Ann Clin Psychiatry 1999;11:55–59.
36 Baldassano CF, Marangell LB, Gyulai L, et al: Gender differences in bipolar disorder: retrospective data from the first 500 STEP-BD participants. Bipolar Disord 2005;7:465–470.
37 Wildes JE, Marcus MD, Fagiolini A: Obesity in patients with bipolar disorder: a biopsychosocial-behavioral model. J Clin Psychiatry 2006;67:904–915.
38 Franks S: Polycystic ovary syndrome. N Engl J Med 1995;333:853–861.
39 Dunaif A, Thomas A: Current concepts in the polycystic ovary syndrome. Annu Rev Med 2001;52:401–419.
40 Dockerty MB, Jackson RL: The Stein-Leventhal syndrome: analysis of 43 cases with special reference to association with endometrial carcinoma. Am J Obstet Gynecol 1957;73:161–173.
41 Carmina E, Lobo RA: Polycystic ovary syndrome (PCOS): arguably the most common endocrinopathy is associated with significant morbidity in women. J Clin Endocrinol Metab 1999;84:1897–1899.
42 Hopkinson ZE, Sattar N, Fleming R, Greer IA: Polycystic ovarian syndrome: the metabolic syndrome comes to gynaecology. BMJ 1998;317:329–332.
43 Pasquali R, Casimirri F: The impact of obesity on hyperandrogenism and polycystic ovary syndrome in premenopausal women. Clin Endocrinol (Oxf) 1993;39:1–16.
44 Kirchengast S, Huber J: Body composition characteristics and body fat distribution in lean women with polycystic ovary syndrome. Hum Reprod 2001;16:1255–1260.
45 Carmina E, Bucchieri S, Esposito A, et al: Abdominal fat quantity and distribution in women with polycystic ovary syndrome and extent of its relation to insulin resistance. J Clin Endocrinol Metab 2007;92:2500–2505.
46 Third Report of the National Cholesterol Education Program (NCEP) Expert Panel on Detection, Evaluation, and Treatment of High Blood Cholesterol in Adults (Adult Treatment Panel III) final report. Circulation 2002;106:3143–3421.
47 Larsson B, Bengtsson C, Bjorntorp P, et al: Is abdominal body fat distribution a major explanation for the sex difference in the incidence of myocardial infarction? The study of men born in 1913 and the study of women, Goteborg, Sweden. Am J Epidemiol 1992;135:266–273.
48 Wild RA, Alaupovic P, Parker IJ: Lipid and apolipoprotein abnormalities in hirsute women. I. The association with insulin resistance. Am J Obstet Gynecol 1992;166:1191–1196; discussion 1196–1197.
49 Legro RS, Blanche P, Krauss RM, Lobo RA: Alterations in low-density lipoprotein and high-density lipoprotein subclasses among Hispanic women with polycystic ovary syndrome: influence of insulin and genetic factors. Fertil Steril 1999;72:990–995.
50 Tiras MB, Yalcin R, Noyan V, et al: Alterations in cardiac flow parameters in patients with polycystic ovarian syndrome. Hum Reprod 1999;14:1949–1952.
51 Paradisi G, Steinberg HO, Hempfling A, et al: Polycystic ovary syndrome is associated with endothelial dysfunction. Circulation 2001;103:1410–1415.
52 Orio F Jr, Palomba S, Spinelli L, et al: The cardiovascular risk of young women with polycystic ovary syndrome: an observational, analytical, prospective case-control study. J Clin Endocrinol Metab 2004;89:3696–3701.
53 Vural B, Caliskan E, Turkoz E, Kilic T, Demirci A: Evaluation of metabolic syndrome frequency and premature carotid atherosclerosis in young women with polycystic ovary syndrome. Hum Reprod 2005;20:2409–2413.
54 Diamanti-Kandarakis E, Piperi C, Spina J, et al: Polycystic ovary syndrome: the influence of environmental and genetic factors. Hormones (Athens) 2006;5:17–34.
55 Luef G, Abraham I, Haslinger M, et al: Polycystic ovaries, obesity and insulin resistance in women with epilepsy: a comparative study of carbamazepine and valproic acid in 105 women. J Neurol 2002;249:835–841.
56 Isojarvi JI, Laatikainen TJ, Pakarinen AJ, Juntunen KT, Myllyla VV: Polycystic ovaries and hyperandrogenism in women taking valproate for epilepsy. N Engl J Med 1993;329:1383–1388.
57 O'Donovan C, Kusumakar V, Graves GR, Bird DC: Menstrual abnormalities and polycystic ovary syndrome in women taking valproate for bipolar mood disorder. J Clin Psychiatry 2002;63:322–330.
58 McIntyre RS, Mancini DA, McCann S, Srinivasan J, Kennedy SH: Valproate, bipolar disorder and polycystic ovarian syndrome. Bipolar Disord 2003;5:28–35.

59 Joffe H, Cohen LS, Suppes T, et al: Valproate is associated with new-onset oligoamenorrhea with hyperandrogenism in women with bipolar disorder. Biol Psychiatry 2006;59:1078–1086.

60 Joffe H, Cohen LS, Suppes T, et al: Longitudinal follow-up of reproductive and metabolic features of valproate-associated polycystic ovarian syndrome features: a preliminary report. Biol Psychiatry 2006; 60:1378–1381.

61 Sit D: Women and bipolar disorder across the life span. J Am Med Womens Assoc 2004;59:91–100.

62 Kupka RW, Nolen WA, Post RM, et al: High rate of autoimmune thyroiditis in bipolar disorder: lack of association with lithium exposure. Biol Psychiatry 2002;51:305–311.

63 Kusalic M, Engelsmann F: Effect of lithium maintenance therapy on thyroid and parathyroid function. J Psychiatry Neurosci 1999;24:227–233.

64 Peselow E, Dunner D, Fieve R: Lithium Carbonate and Weight Gain. J Affect Disorder 1980;2:303–310.

65 Bowden C, Calabrese J, McElroy S: A randomized, placebo-controlled 12-month trial of divalproex and lithium in treatment of outpatients with bipolar I disorder. Divalproex Maintenance Study Group. Arch Gen Psychiatry 2000;57:481–489.

66 Vestergaard P, Amdisen A, Schou M: Clinically significant side effects of lithium treatment. Acta Psychiatr Scand 1980;62:193–200.

67 Garland E, Remick R, Zis A: Weight gain with antidepressants and lithium. J Clin Psychopharmacology 1998;8:323–330.

68 Vendsborg P, Bach-Mortensen M, Rafaelson O: Fat cell number and weight gain in lithium treated patients. Acta Psychiatr Scand 1976a;53:355–359.

69 Aronne L, Segal K: Weight gain in the treatment of mood disorders. J Clin Psychiatry 2003;64(suppl 8):22–30.

70 Baptista T, Teneud L, Contreras Q: Lithium and body weight gain. Pharmacopsychiatry 1995;28:35–44.

71 Levine S, Saltzman A: Lithium increases gastrointestinal tract weight of male or female rats but it increases body weight only in females. Prog Neuropsychopharmacol Biol Psychiatry 2008;32:29–33.

72 Vendsborg P, Rafaelson O: Lithium in man: effect on glucose intolerance and serum electrolytes. Acta Psychiatr Scand 1973;49:601–610.

73 Plenges P, Mellerup E, Rafaelson O: Lithium action on glycogen synthesis in rat brain, liver and diaphragm. J Psychiatr Res 1970;8:29–36.

74 Mellerup E, Thomson H, Bjorun N: Lithium, weight gain and serum insulin in manic-depressive patients. Acta Psychiatr Scand 1972;48:332–336.

75 van der Velde C, Gordon M: Manic-depressive illness, diabetes mellitus, and lithium carbonate. Arch Gen Psychiatry 1969;21:478–485.

76 Vieweg W, Godleski L, Hundley P, Yank G: Lithium, polyuria and abnormal diurnal weight gain in psychosis. Acta Psychiatr Scand 1988;78:510–514.

77 Saran A: Antidiabetic Effects of Lithium. J Clin Psychiatry 1982;43:383–384.

78 Baranyi A, Yazdani R, Haas-Krammer A, Stepan A: Atypical antipsychotics and metabolic syndrome. Wien Med Wochenschr 2007;157:255–270.

79 Elmslie J, Mann J, Silverstone J: Determinants of overweight and obesity in patients with bipolar disorder. J Clin Psychiatry 2001;62:486–491.

80 Newcomer J: Second-generation (atypical) antipsychotics and metabolic effects. CNS Drugs 2005; 19(suppl 1):1–93.

81 Baptista T, De Mendoza S, Beaulieu S, Bermudez A, Martinez M: The metabolic syndrome during atypical antipsychotic drug treatment: mechanisms and management. Metab Syndr Relat Disord 2004;2:290–307.

82 Newcomer J, Haupt D, Fucetola R, et al: Abnormalities in glucose regulation during antipsychotic treatment of schizophrenia. Arch Gen Psychiatry 2002;59:337–345.

83 Bergman R, Ader M: Atypical antipsychotics and glucose homeostasis. J Clin Psychiatry 2005;66:504–514.

84 Albaugh VL, Henry CR, Bello NT, et al: Hormonal and metabolic effects of olanzapine and clozapine related to body weight in rodents. Obesity (Silver Spring) 2006;14:36–51.

85 Birkenaes A, Birkeland K, Engh J, Farden A: Dyslipidemia independent of body mass in antipsychotic-treated patients under real-life conditions. J Clin Psychopharmacology 2008;28:132–137.

86 Olfson M, Marcus S, Corey-Lisle P, Tuomari A, Hines P, L'Italien G: Hyperlipidemia following treatment with antipsychotic medications. Am J Psychiatry 2006;163:1821–1825.

87 Vestri H, Maianu L, Moellering D, Garvey W: Atypical antipsychotic drugs directly impair insulin action in adipocytes: effects on glucose transport, lipogenesis, and antilipolysis. Neuropsychopharmacology 2007;32:765–772.

88 Richards AA, Hickman IJ, Wang AY, et al: Olanzapine treatment is associated with reduced high molecular weight adiponectin in serum: a potential mechanism for olanzapine-induced insulin resistance in patients with schizophrenia. J Clin Psychopharmacol 2006;26:232–237.

89 Baptista T, Kin NM, Beaulieu S, de Baptista EA: Obesity and related metabolic abnormalities during antipsychotic drug administration: mechanisms, management and research perspectives. Pharmacopsychiatry 2002;35:205–219.

90 Rubi B, Ljubicić S, Pournourmohammadi S: Dopamine D2-like receptors are expressed in pancreatic beta cells and mediate inhibition of insulin secretion. J Biol Chem 2005;280:36824–36832.
91 Palik E, Birkas K, Faludi G: Correlation of serum ghrelin levels with body mass index and carbohydrate metabolism in patients treated with atypical antipsychotics. Diabetes Res Clin Pract 2005; 68(suppl 1):S60–S64.
92 Sporn A, Bobb A, Gogtay N: Hormonal correlates of clozapine-induced weight gain in psychotic children: an exploratory study. J Am Acad Child Adolesc Psychiatry 2005;44:925–933.
93 Togo T, Hasegawa K, Miura S: Serum ghrelin concentrations in patients receiving olanzapine or risperidone. Psychopharmacology 2004;172:230–232.
94 Theisen F, Gebhardt S, Bromel T: A prospective study of serum ghrelin levels in patients treated with clozapine. J Neural Transm 2005;112:1411–1416.
95 Wang PW, Ketter TA: Clinical use of carbamazepine for bipolar disorders. Expert Opin Pharmacother 2005;6:2887–2902.
96 Steinhoff BJ: Optimizing therapy of seizures in patients with endocrine disorders. Neurology 2006;67(suppl 4):S23–S27.
97 Kim JY, Lee HW: Metabolic and hormonal disturbances in women with epilepsy on antiepileptic drug monotherapy. Epilepsia 2007;48:1366–1370.
98 Zarzar MN, Graham J, Roberts J, Thompson T, Nanry K: Effectiveness and weight effects of open-label lamotrigine with and without concomitant psychotropic medications in patients with bipolar I disorder. MedGenMed 2007;9:41.
99 Ben-Menachem E: Weight issues for people with epilepsy: a review. Epilepsia 2007;48(suppl 9):42–45.
100 Khanna V, Arumugam S, Roy S, Mittra S, Bansal VS: Topiramate and type 2 diabetes: an old wine in a new bottle. Expert Opin Ther Targets 2008;12:81–90.
101 Tata AL, Kockler DR: Topiramate for binge-eating disorder associated with obesity. Ann Pharmacother 2006;40:1993–1997.
102 Post RM, Altshuler LL, Frye MA, et al: New findings from the Bipolar Collaborative Network: clinical implications for therapeutics. Curr Psychiatry Rep 2006;8:489–497.

Mytilee P. Vemuri, MD, MBA
Stanford University, Department of Psychiatry
401 Quarry Road
Stanford, CA 94305 (USA)
Tel. +1 650 725–1774, Fax +1 650 724–9900, E-mail mvemuri@stanford.edu

Thakore J, Leonard BE (eds): Metabolic Effects of Psychotropic Drugs.
Mod Trends Pharmacopsychiatry. Basel, Karger, 2009, vol 26, pp 25–46

Obesity and Mental Illness[1]

Leslie Citrome[a] · Betty Vreeland[b]

[a]New York University School of Medicine, Department of Psychiatry, and the Nathan S. Kline Institute for Psychiatric Research, Orangeburg, N.Y.; [b]University Behavioral HealthCare, the School of Nursing, and the Departments of Psychiatry and Family Medicine, Robert Wood Johnson Medical School, University of Medicine and Dentistry of New Jersey, Piscataway, N.J., USA

Abstract

Obesity is one of the most common physical health care problems among persons with severe and persistent mental illness. Obesity is a complex multifactorial chronic disease that develops from the interaction between genotype and the environment. Among individuals with serious mental illnesses, an unhealthy lifestyle, as well as the effects of psychotropic medications, such as second-generation antipsychotics, can contribute to the development of this problem. Excess body weight increases the risk for many medical problems, including type 2 diabetes mellitus, coronary heart disease, osteoarthritis, hypertension, and gallbladder disease. Monitoring body weight is essential, and weight gain early in treatment can help predict those at high risk for substantial weight gain. Children, adolescents, and first-episode patients are at higher risk for weight gain. Lifestyle therapies and other non-pharmacological interventions have been shown to be effective in controlled clinical trials, but the evidence base for adjunctive medication strategies such as with orlistat, sibutramine, amantadine, nizatidine, metformin, topiramate, and others, is conflicting. Switching antipsychotic medication may or may not be clinically feasible, but can lead to a reduction in body weight. At the very least, a 'small steps approach' to managing weight should be offered to all patients who are started on second generation antipsychotics.

Obesity is a complex multifactorial chronic disease that develops from the interaction between genotype and the environment. Obesity in individuals with mental disorders such as schizophrenia has been attributed to various factors, including a sedentary lifestyle, poor nutritional choices or lack of access to healthy foods, the effects of both the mental disorder itself and the medications used to treat it, and lack of access to adequate preventative medical care. Excess body weight increases the risk for many medical problems, including type 2 diabetes mellitus, coronary heart disease, osteoarthritis, hypertension, and gallbladder disease [1]. Abdominal or visceral obesity is

[1] Portions of this chapter have been adapted with kind permission from: Citrome L, Vreeland B: Schizophrenia, obesity, and antipsychotic medications: what can we do? Postgrad Med 2008;120(2):18–33.

particularly associated with increased risk for insulin resistance and/or the metabolic syndrome and for type 2 diabetes mellitus [2], and persons with schizophrenia have greater visceral adiposity than healthy individuals [3].

The clinical problem of obesity has become more apparent with the availability of second-generation, or 'atypical', antipsychotics. Their advantage over the older 'neuroleptics' have principally been in their lower propensity for extrapyramidal side effects, including tremor, rigidity, and akathisia [4]. However, one of the most troubling adverse effects of the second-generation antipsychotics is treatment-associated weight gain. The second-generation antipsychotics available today differ in their propensity for weight gain and the degree of weight change can also vary from patient to patient. Efficacy may also differ from drug to drug, and patient to patient, making medication selection and monitoring for weight gain a complex issue and can give rise to significant therapeutic dilemmas. Moreover, obesity can be an obstacle to adherence to medication, as evidenced by a mail survey of persons with schizophrenia where BMI status and subjective distress from weight gain were predictors of noncompliance [5].

This chapter addresses what the clinician can do to ameliorate the problem of overweight and obesity observed in patients with mental disorders, particularly schizophrenia. When using antipsychotics, especially those most associated with weight gain, ongoing monitoring is essential. Certain patients, such as children, adolescents, and those with their first episode of schizophrenia, are at higher risk for weight gain, even when using the second-generation antipsychotic medications that are ordinarily considered as 'weight-neutral'. Early monitoring can identify early weight gainers; these patients are at significant risk for substantial weight gain. Lifestyle interventions are crucial when weight gain occurs and switching antipsychotic medication is not a viable option. Adjunctive medications for weight loss can be considered but randomized clinical trials for this intervention have generally not been encouraging.

Definitions

Body mass index (BMI), calculated as the quotient of body weight (kg) divided by the square of height (m), is commonly used to assess body weight. On-line calculators for BMI are readily available (for example, the website from the Centers for Disease Control and Prevention, http://www.cdc.gov/nccdphp/dnpa/bmi/calc-bmi). Overweight is defined as a BMI between 25 and 29.9 inclusive, and obesity is defined as having a BMI of 30 or greater. BMI-related health risks are well established, with health risk considered 'high' for BMI of 30–34.9, 'very high' for BMI 35–39.9, and 'extremely high' for BMI greater than 40 [6].

Alternate definitions have focused on waist-to-hip ratios or waist circumference used in the definitions for metabolic syndrome developed by the World Health Organization and the National Cholesterol Education Program Expert Panel on

Detection, Evaluation, and Treatment of High Blood Cholesterol in Adults (NCEP), respectively [7].

Moreover, these definitions may not apply in all ethnic groups. For example, waist circumference for Asians is generally lower, requiring a lower cut-off of 90 cm in men (instead of 102 cm in the NCEP definition) or 80 cm in women (instead of 88 cm), when assessing the prevalence of central obesity [8]. In Japan, the definition of obesity is a BMI of at least 25, rather than the 30 used among Caucasians [9].

Quantitative measures of body fat have been developed, notably dual energy X-ray absorptiometry (DEXA) [10].

Epidemiology

Obesity has reached epidemic proportions in the general population. Current International Obesity Task Force estimates suggest that at least 1.1 billion adults are overweight including 312 million who are obese; this represents a doubling and trebling in less than two decades [11]. Among randomly selected middle-aged participants from 34 populations in 21 countries from the early 1980s to the mid-1990s, mean BMI as well as the prevalence of overweight increased in virtually all Western European countries, Australia, the USA, and China, and was related to increasing trends in total energy supply per capita [12]. Since 1980, the prevalence of obesity in Great Britain in adults has almost trebled with obesity prevalence in 2002 of 23% for men and 25% for women [13]. In the US, obesity prevalence among adults in 2003–2004 was 32%, and the prevalence of extreme obesity (BMI of at least 40) was 2.8% in men and 6.9% in women [14].

Patients with schizophrenia have higher rates of obesity [15]. Among the patients participating in phase 1 of the randomized and double-blinded 18-month Clinical Antipsychotic Trials of Intervention Effectiveness schizophrenia study (CATIE), the mean BMI was 30 [16]. Moreover, waist circumference exceeded norms for 46% of all subjects (n = 1435), 37% of all men (n = 1059), 73% of all women (n = 376), 48% of all Caucasians (n = 858), 43% of all Blacks (n = 504), and 47% of all Hispanics (n = 167).

Contributory Factors

Overweight and obesity is related to a mismatch between energy intake, expenditure, and storage [17]. A sedentary lifestyle associated with increased intake of high caloric food will lead to increased weight. For example, about 7,800 kcal of chemical energy is contained in 1 kg of adipose tissue so that even a small increase in intake (such as 0.5 liters a day of a sugared carbonated beverage or 200 kcal) can lead to a significant amount of weight gain of 9 kg in one year if these additional calories are not expended but instead stored as fat. The availability of different foods and the amount consumed

Table 1. What the world eats (compiled from [18])

Country	Meat consumption (kg per person per year)	Obesity prevalence men, women , %	Life expectancy, men, women, years
Australia	107	21, 23	78, 83
Bhutan	3	5, 13	60, 62
Bosnia	21	14, 22	69, 76
Chad	14	0.3, 1	46, 49
China	52	1, 1.5	70, 73
Cuba	32	12, 21	75, 79
Ecuador	45	6, 15	68, 74
Egypt	22	22, 39	65, 69
France	101	7, 6	76, 84
Germany	82 (30 in sausages)	20, 19	76, 82
Great Britain	80	19, 21	76, 81
Greenland	114	16, 22	64, 70
Guatemala	24	13, 25	63, 69
India	5	0.9, 1.1	60, 62
Italy	90	12, 12	77, 83
Japan	44	2, 2	78, 85
Kuwait	60	30, 49	76, 77
Mali	19	0.4, 3	44, 46
Mexico	59	20, 32	72, 77
Mongolia	109	5, 25	60, 66
Philippines	31	1, 3	72, 65
Poland	78	13, 18	71, 79
Turkey	19	11, 32	68, 72
USA	125	32, 38	75, 80

varies from country to country. Table 1 outlines meat consumption, prevalence of obesity, and life expectancy for 24 different countries [18].

Patients with mental disorders such as schizophrenia may make poor dietary choices [19]. In patients with an increased risk for central adiposity to begin with [3], this combination of poor diet and lack of physical activity is particularly problematic.

Psychotropic medications such as antipsychotics [4], antidepressants [20], and anticonvulsants [21], have been associated with weight gain. It is not uncommon for these medications to be used in combination. Possible mechanisms for medication-associated weight gain include weight loss before drug treatment, food craving, alteration in resting metabolic rate, sedation/decreased physical activity, change in neurotransmitters (in general, alpha-adrenergic neurotransmission is thought to stimulate appetite, whereas beta-adrenergic, histaminergic, dopaminergic, and sero-

Table 2. Weight change in phase 1 of the Clinical Antipsychotic Trials of Antipsychotic Effectiveness for Schizophrenia trial [26]

Antipsychotic	Mean weight change kg/month	Median weight change kg/month	5th and 95th percentile weight change, kg/month
Olanzapine	+0.909	+0.363	−0.636, +4.32
Quetiapine	+0.227	+0.045	−2.00, +2.86
Risperidone	+0.182	0	−2.09, +2.59
Perphenazine	−0.091	−0.045	−2.23, +1.82
Ziprasidone	−0.136	−0.136	−2.41, +2.58

toninergic signal transduction confers satiety) and alteration of neuropeptides such as leptin and cytokines such as tumor necrosis factor [22].

Second-Generation Antipsychotics

Second-generation antipsychotics are a major source of concern regarding weight gain. Attempts have been made to identify specific receptor-binding profiles of antipsychotics to aid in the prediction of propensity for weight gain [23], however there is much individual variation, and most of the information available at present comes from clinical observations. In a comprehensive meta-analysis of weight change after 10 weeks of treatment at a standard dose of antipsychotics, mean increases in body weight were calculated for the different medications [24]. Clozapine and olanzapine had the largest weight gains with 4.45 and 4.15 kg, respectively. Risperidone was associated with a more modest 2.10 kg gain. Ziprasidone appeared essentially weight neutral with a mean gain of 0.04 kg. Insufficient data were available to evaluate quetiapine at 10 weeks, but subsequent studies have indicated that quetiapine also has a moderate to high propensity toward gain, particularly over the long term, as demonstrated in a prospective, naturalistic study [25]. Aripiprazole, the newest second-generation antipsychotic medication to become commercially available, is generally considered to be weight neutral.

Examining mean weight change as observed in clinical trials is not always informative as to how often this actually will be encountered in clinical practice. There is large individual variability regarding weight gain, even with agents commonly thought of as being inexorably tied to obesity. In the CATIE study weight change per month of antipsychotic treatment was reported both in terms of mean change and in terms of median and range [26]. Table 2 demonstrates that although mean weight change followed the expected pattern, some patients randomized to olanzapine lost 0.64 kg per month, and some gained 4.3 kg per month. Patients randomized to weight neutral medications still show variability in weight change, with some patients randomized to ziprasidone losing 2.4 kg per month and others gaining 2.7 lb per month. Weight gain greater than 7% from baseline to last observation occurred among 30% of the patients randomized to olanzapine, 16% for quetiapine, 14% for risperidone, 12% for perphenazine, and 7% for ziprasidone. Number needed to treat (NNT) to encounter one additional case of weight gain greater than 7% when using olanzapine versus perphenazine (a first-generation antipsychotic) was 6, versus quetiapine 8, versus risperidone 7, and versus ziprasidone 5 [27]. This means for every 5 patients randomized to olanzapine instead of ziprasidone, there was one additional case of a patient on olanzapine gaining greater than 7% of their initial body weight. Keeping in mind patients randomized to olanzapine had a longer mean time on medication than the other antipsychotics, and thus had a greater opportunity to accumulate weight, these single-digit NNTs nevertheless represent clinically significant differences [28].

Switching antipsychotics can lead to weight loss. Ultimately, there will need to be a favorable balance of benefit to risk [29]. Deciding whether to continue treatment with a particular antipsychotic or switch the patient to another can pose substantial dilemmas for the clinician. The choice to 'switch or stay' is a highly individualized decision. Evidence-based medicine philosophy states that relevant clinical trials can inform the clinician in making thoughtful individualized treatment decisions but there are no guarantees of weight gain or loss or drug efficacy. With these caveats, consideration should be given to switching to a more weight-neutral medication when encountering rapid weight gain with a particular antipsychotic. For example, in the CATIE study, of 61 patients who gained over 7% of their body weight in phase 1, 42% of ziprasidone-treated patients, 20% of risperidone-treated patients, 7% of quetiapine-treated patients, and 0% of olanzapine-treated patients lost over 7% of their body weight during phase 2 [30]. The NNT to encounter one additional case of weight loss greater than 7% when using ziprasidone versus olanzapine or quetiapine was 3, and versus risperidone 5 [29]. The findings from CATIE are consistent with earlier reports from open-label studies, such as a post-hoc analysis of a 20-week study where switching from olanzapine to risperidone resulted in a reduction of prevalence of metabolic syndrome in overweight or obese patients, including reductions in body weight and BMI [31]. In another report of 3 studies in which outpatients experiencing were switched to 6 weeks of open-label ziprasidone, patients switched from olanzapine experienced a mean weight loss of 1.76 kg, those switched from risperidone had a lesser reduction in weight (–0.86 kg), and those switched from first-generation antipsychotics had a non-significant increase (+0.27 kg) [32]. In an 8-week study where patients were switched from other antipsychotics to open-label aripiprazole (92% were receiving olanzapine or risperidone prior to the switch), the mean weight loss from baseline ranged from 1.3 kg to 1.7 kg, the incidence of weight loss of at least 7% of total body weight ranged from 7% to 15%, and the incidence of weight gain of at least 7% of total body weight ranged from 3% to 5%, depending on the switching technique [33].

Early weight gain may be predictive of future substantial weight gain. One can use the time course for weight gain with olanzapine for early identification of those at risk before substantial weight gain has occurred [34, 35]. Patients taking olanzapine who gain 5% or more of their body weight within the first 4–12 weeks of treatment and who are going to remain on olanzapine will require more active behavioral and/or pharmacologic interventions than patients who gain weight more slowly or not at all. Although weight gain may plateau after 40 weeks or so, by that time one-half of patients receiving olanzapine will have gained up to 10 kg, and some substantially more than that [36]. The pattern of weight gain with quetiapine is also consistent with the idea that it can occur early (within 12 weeks) [37]. Within the approved range, antipsychotic dose does not appear to be predictive of weight gain for olanzapine [36] but there may be differences at higher-than-approved doses [38]. For risperidone, in a short (6-week) trial, higher doses were associated with more weight gain [39]. Data regarding a dose relationship with weight gain with quetiapine is conflicting [37, 40]. Low initial BMI (<25) may be a predictor of some future weight gain in some patients with any of the second-generation antipsychotic medications.

Children and adolescents [41], and patients in their first episode of psychosis may be at heightened risk for weight gain with antipsychotic medication [42]. In a 52-week randomized double-blind clinical trial in patients early in their course of psychotic illness, 80% of patients in the olanzapine group, 50% in the quetiapine group, and 58% in the risperidone group, gained at least 7% of their baseline weight at week 52 [43]. Similarly, in the 1-year European First-Episode Schizophrenia Trial, weight gain greater than 7% from baseline was observed in 86% of the patients randomized to olanzapine, 65% for those on quetiapine, 37% for those on ziprasidone, and 53% for those on haloperidol [44]. Amisulpride, an antipsychotic not commercialized in the USA, was associated with a rate of 63% on this outcome.

Monitoring of patients receiving psychotropic medications for weight and metabolic parameters is crucial. The report from the Consensus Development Conference on Antipsychotic Drugs and Obesity and Diabetes Consensus Panel contains valuable advice for appropriate and prudent monitoring [45]. The most frequently assessed parameter in the recommendations is weight. At a minimum it is obtained at baseline, monthly for the first 3 months, and then quarterly. However, monitoring weight at each and every patient visit will allow the clinician to catch a problem early, before substantial weight gain has set in, and underscore to both the patient and the clinician the importance of physical fitness. Additionally, patients and/or caregivers can be educated about monitoring weight and report back to the clinician.

Lifestyle Therapies and Other Nonpharmacological Interventions

Maintaining a normal weight, even without the additional challenges frequently associated with mental illness, is difficult for most individuals. There is a commonly held belief that persons with schizophrenia cannot make lifestyle changes that improve ones' health such as choosing to eat healthier, becoming more physically active, and achieving significant weight loss. However, research in the form of controlled clinical trials as listed in table 3 suggests that people with schizophrenia are able to benefit from lifestyle interventions that promote weight maintenance and weight loss [46–61]. Additionally, the report from the Consensus Development Conference on Antipsychotic Drugs and Obesity and Diabetes Consensus Panel recommends that in addition to monitoring nutrition and physical activity counseling be provided for all patients who are overweight or obese, particularly if they are starting treatment with a second-generation antipsychotic that is associated with significant weight gain [45]. Therefore, it is important that clinicians working with individuals with serious mental illnesses to become familiar with lifestyle interventions that address weight. This section provides a brief overview of lifestyle interventions recommended by the National Institutes of Health (NIH) in the general population, reviews the available data on lifestyle and other nonpharmacologic weight management strategies in people with serious mental illnesses, and makes suggestions for how to utilize these interventions in clinical care.

The *Practical Guide: Identification, Evaluation, and Treatment of Overweight and Obesity in Adults* from NIH describes how health care practitioners can provide individuals with evidence-based information and the support needed to effectively lose weight and keep it down [62]. Treatment of overweight and obesity is considered a two-step process which includes assessment and management. Prevention of weight gain with lifestyle therapy is indicated in any patient with a BMI of ≥25; and weight loss for any patient who has a BMI of ≥30, or a BMI of 25–29.9 or waist circumference >88 cm (women) or >102 cm (men) *and* ≥2 risk factors including cigarette smoking, hypertension, high low-density lipoprotein (LDL ≥160 mg/dl), low high-density lipoprotein (HDL <35/mg/dl), impaired fasting glucose (between 100 and 125 mg/dl), family history of premature coronary heart disease, age ≥45 for males and ≥55 for women, and physical inactivity. Patients at very high absolute risk including established coronary heart disease (CHD) and other atherosclerotic diseases (such as a history of myocardial infarction and angina pectoris), type 2 diabetes, and sleep apnea need to be identified and their conditions appropriated managed. Additionally, other obesity-associated diseases including gynecological abnormalities, osteoarthritis, gallstones and stress incontinence, need to be identified and treated. The guide notes that the decision to lose weight must be made jointly by the clinician and the patient and that the person may chose as a goal not to lose weight but rather to prevent further weight gain. The guide further suggests that the clinician determine the individuals' 'readiness' to make lifestyle changes. There are three major components of weight loss therapy described which are collectively referred to as 'lifestyle therapies': (1) dietary therapy, (2) increased physical activity, and (3) behavior therapy. Examples of behavioral strategies include self-monitoring, stress management, stimulus control, problem solving, contingency management, cognitive restructuring and social support. If lifestyle therapy is initiated, it should be attempted for at least 6 months before considering pharmacotherapy, and it should be tailored to the needs of the individual. The guide states that persons with an 'uncontrolled' serious mental illness, for whom caloric restriction might exacerbate the illness, should be excluded from weight loss therapy. No specific information is provided about how to adapt lifestyle therapies for people with mental illnesses that are not 'uncontrolled'. However, a 'small steps approach' to weight maintenance and weight loss, which is mentioned later in this section, may be particularly helpful for people with serious mental illnesses. The reader is referred to the actual guide itself for more in-depth information about how to assess and manage weight problems.

Research suggests that most self-directed and commercial programs that teach lifestyle modifications induce reductions of up to 5% of initial weight [63]. While the body of evidence is not as vast as that in the general population, research findings suggests that when people with schizophrenia participate in lifestyle and other nonpharmacologic weight management interventions there is a significant improvement in weight (table 3).

Controlled trials comparing nonpharmacologic interventions designed to address weight problems in people with serious mental illnesses are methodologically varied [46–61]. Most nonpharmacologic interventions studied emphasize dietary and other lifestyle changes. They vary in their approach from cognitive-behavioral interventions, to commercial programs, to manualized psychoeducational wellness programs. They also differ in terms of duration, number of sessions, and amount of weight loss reported.

A study by Dansinger et al. [64] assessed adherence rates and effectiveness of 4 popular diets (Atkins©, Zone©, Weight Watchers©, and Ornish©) as a part of individualized weight control strategies in 160 overweight adults without mental illness. After 1 year, overall adherence rates (i.e. those who completed the study) ranged from 50 to 65%, with a mean weight loss among the 4 diet groups ranging from 2.1 to 3.3 kg. In contrast, the 'Healthy Living' program [53] studied adherence and weight loss in overweight and obese subjects with schizophrenia or schizoaffective disorder who had gained weight on various second-generation antipsychotics. This was a nonrandomized study where 31 subjects participated in a 52-week lifestyle intervention entitled 'Healthy Living' and 20 subjects received 'treatment as usual'. The Healthy Living program consisted of nutrition, exercise, and behavioral interventions and was designed to assist individuals with schizophrenia who had gained weight to make small long-lasting lifestyle changes that would have a positive effect on weight loss and overall health. At 1 year, the mean adherence (attendance) rate was 69% and a mean weight loss of 3.7 kg in study completers. In comparison with the Dansinger data [64], the subjects with schizophrenia not only had similar adherence rates, but also demonstrated greater weight loss than subjects without schizophrenia. Additionally, the Healthy Living study, found that subjects who received the intervention had a 3.0% weight reduction compared with a 3.5% weight gain with 'treatment as usual'.

Another lifestyle intervention that has had success in managing weight in people with serious mental illness is the 'Solutions for Wellness' program which is free

Table 3. Controlled clinical trials of nonpharmacological interventions for weight gain among patients with schizophrenia

Author	Active intervention	Antipsychotic received (and other qualifications)	Study length weeks	n	Helpful?	Weight change observed in intervention group (vs. control group)
Harmatz [46]	behavior modification in which money is lost for failure to lose weight or group therapy or diet only	not reported (all overweight; hospitalized 5 to 7 years with schizophrenia)	6 (+4 follow-up)	21	yes	–6.8 kg (vs. little or no change in group therapy or diet only groups)
Wu [47]	diet and regular physical activity per protocol	clozapine (and BMI >27)	26	53	yes	–4.2 kg (vs. +1.0 kg)
Mauri [48]	psychoeducational program including diet and use of a pedometer	olanzapine (and an increase in BMI of at least 7%)	24	33	yes	–4.5 kg (vs. no change without the intervention)
Alvarez-Jiménez [49]	early behavioral intervention including behavioral interventions, nutrition, and exercise	drug-naive first-episode psychosis patients started on olanzapine, risperidone, or haloperidol	12	61	yes	+4.1 kg (vs. +6.9 kg); number experiencing weight gain greater than 7% was 39.3% (vs. 78.8%)
Littrell [50]	intervention group with psycho-education classes focused on nutrition, exercise, and living a healthy lifestyle	switched to olanzapine at start of study	16 (26)	70	yes	–0.03 kg (vs. +4.3 kg)
Evans [51]	nutrition education sessions	olanzapine (started within 12 weeks)	26	51	yes	+2.0 kg (vs. +6.0 kg); number experiencing weight gain greater than 7% was 13% (vs. 64%)
Vreeland [52][a] Menza [53][a]	nutrition, exercise, and behavioral interventions	olanzapine, risperidone, clozapine, quetiapine	12 (52)	31 (51)	yes	–3.0 kg (vs +3.2 kg)
Ball [54][a]	weight watchers and offered supervised exercise sessions	olanzapine (and who had gained at least 7% of their pretreatment body weight)	10	11 (22)	maybe	–2.3 kg (vs. –0.2 kg), but this was only significant for men and not women
Brar [55]	behavioral treatment	risperidone (switched from olanzapine and with a BMI > 26)	14	72	maybe	–2.0 kg (vs. –1.1 kg) but not statistically significant
Kwon [56]	education, diet, and exercise management	olanzapine (and an increase in weight of at least 7%)	12	48	yes	–3.94 kg (vs. –1.48 kg)
Weber [57]	cognitive/behavioral group intervention, modified after the Diabetes Prevention Project program	olanzapine, risperidone, ziprasidone, quetiapine (and BMI of at least 25 and impaired glucose tolerance)	16	15	maybe	–2.4 kg (vs. –0.6 kg) but not statistically significant

Table 3. Continued

Author	Active intervention	Antipsychotic received (and other qualifications)	Study length weeks	n	Helpful?	Weight change observed in intervention group (vs. control group)
Khazaal [58]	cognitive and behavioural treatment	olanzapine, risperidone, clozapine, quetiapine, amisulpride, first-generation antipsychotic (and weight gain af at least 2 kg)	24	61	yes	–3.5 kg (vs. +1.7 kg)
Brown [59]	six weekly health promotion sessions	not reported	6	28	maybe	–0.40 kg (vs. +1.11 kg)
McKibbin [60]	diabetes awareness and rehabilitation training	any (and age over 40 years and with diabetes mellitus)	24	64	yes	–2.3 kg (vs. +2.7 kg)
Rotatori [61]	behavioral self-control program	not reported	14	14	yes	–3.3 kg (vs. +2.5 kg)

[a] These studies had a comparison group composed of matched controls, rather than a randomized design. The numbers in parentheses represent the total number of subjects reported for both the intervention and comparison groups.

(sponsored by Eli Lilly and Company) and available in two formats: the 'personalized' program and the 'manualized' program. The Solutions for Wellness personalized program was evaluated in a study of 7,188 patients with mental illness, 83% of who were obese or overweight [65]. The 6-month intervention was individualized and used diet, exercise and behavioral strategies. Patients were not required to meet any enrollment criteria, including diagnosis, treatment, weight, or risk for weight gain. The mean change in weight was –2.77 kg and the mean change in BMI was –0.93.

In addition, there is also a Solutions for Wellness manualized program [66], which is a free, manualized, psychoeducational wellness program designed to inspire and assist persons with mental illness to choose healthier eating and physical activity patterns. In contrast to the personalized program, which is designed for individuals who are more independent and can benefit from a self-study program, the manualized program was designed to be implemented with the support of health professionals with both groups and individuals. In a quasi-experimental study with 70 patients with schizophrenia or schizoaffective disorder participating in a 4-month intervention which involved a weekly 1-hour psychoeducational intervention using Solutions for Wellness (ed. 2), there was a positive effect on preventing antipsychotic-inducted weight gain as compared to a group who received treatment as usual [50] (table 3).

A 'small steps approach' to weight loss and maintenance may be particularly beneficial to people with serious mental illnesses. Unlike traditional obesity treatment, the goal is prevention of weight gain and modest weight loss over a longer period of time. The approach encourages the use of small everyday changes in dietary and physical activity patterns that people can sustain over time. The small steps approach suggests that trying to achieve some combination of reduced energy intake and increased physical activity that equals approximately 100 kcal/day (such as eliminating one can of a sugared carbonated beverage a day or adding 2,000 steps or about a mile of walking) should prevent weight gain in many adults [67]. A small steps approach was utilized in the Healthy Living study and is incorporated into the Solutions for Wellness (ed. 3) manualized program.

In summary, many of the nonpharmacologic interventions used in the general population may be applicable to adults with major mental disorders. The research on lifestyle and other nonpharmacologic interventions in adults with schizophrenia and schizoaffective disorders indicates that significant weight loss is possible. Programs such as 'Healthy Living' and 'Solutions for Wellness' show promise. Clinicians should provide nutrition and physical activity counseling when starting treatment with a second-generation antipsychotic. At a minimum a 'small steps' approach to counseling patients about lifestyle changes is recommended with referral to more intense programs such as Solutions for Wellness, or more specialized care, such as registered dieticians when 'small steps' fail. More randomized controlled clinical trials are needed in this area.

Pharmacological Interventions

When nonpharmacological interventions fail to control weight gain, and when switching to another antipsychotic has been unsuccessful or is not possible, adjunctive pharmacotherapy may be considered. Drugs that are currently approved by the FDA for the treatment of obesity include orlistat and sibutramine, both of which should be used cautiously with psychotropic medications. These medications should be used only in combination with appropriate diet, exercise, and behavioral programs.

Orlistat is an enteric inhibitor of pancreatic lipase, thus lowering the absorption of dietary fat. Adverse effects include flatulence and steatorrhea if too much fat is consumed. Orlistat was tested for 16 weeks in a randomized, double-blind, placebo-controlled clinical trial in overweight or obese patients treated with clozapine or olanzapine (n = 63, diagnosis not reported) [68]. Adherence to a behavioral program or diet was not required to participate in the study. No statistically significant effect was observed in the whole population, but male patients experienced modest weight loss (–2.36 vs. +0.62 kg on placebo). Weight loss of at least 5% of baseline was observed in 16% of the patients receiving adjunctive orlistat versus 6% receiving placebo (NNT 11, not statistically significant). All 4 patients who discontinued because of diarrhea were receiving orlistat. There is a report that orlistat did not alter bioavailability of haloperidol, clozapine, clomipramine, desipramine, or carbamazepine in 8 patients, however the authors noted the possibility of decreased absorption of concomitantly administered drugs in some individuals, and recommended plasma level monitoring [69].

Sibutramine affects the reuptake of norepinephrine, serotonin and dopamine, and was originally thought to be a potential antidepressant compound, but was ultimately commercialized as a weight loss agent. Sibutramine was tested in a 12-week double-blind, randomized, placebo-controlled study in 37 overweight and obese subjects taking olanzapine for schizophrenia or schizoaffective disorder [70]. For the first 8 weeks all subjects participated in weekly group sessions focused on nutrition and behavioral modification. Although the sibutramine group exhibited a mean increase in systolic blood pressure of 2.1 mm Hg, and presented with a higher rate of anticholinergic side effects and sleep disturbances, greater weight loss was observed at week 12 versus placebo (–3.8 vs. –0.8 kg). A similarly designed study with clozapine conducted among 21 patients by the same research group failed to demonstrate a therapeutic advantage for adjunctive sibutramine [71]. Because sibutramine affects serotonin and norepinephrine reuptake, these two studies [70, 71] excluded patients who received tricyclic, selective serotonin reuptake inhibitor, or monoamine oxidase inhibitor antidepressants in the prior month. When compared with adjunctive topiramate in a 24-week randomized open-label clinical trial, adjunctive sibutramine resulted in similar amounts of weight loss as adjunctive topiramate [72], but generalizability of that study to schizophrenia is limited as the subjects had bipolar disorder and only 35% were receiving antipsychotic medication.

Rimonabant is a cannabinoid antagonist that acts to control appetite and can lead to weight reduction. The proposed indication was to be weight management in people with a BMI of 30, or with a BMI of 27 and at least one comorbid medical condition. However, the manufacturer withdrew its application to sell this agent in the USA amid concerns that it may increase suicidal thinking and depression [73]. There are no published reports of its use in patients with schizophrenia receiving antipsychotics.

Several attempts have been made in managing weight gain with adjunctive therapy utilizing non-FDA approved uses of several classes of medications, including oral hypoglycemics (metformin), anticonvulsants (topiramate), histamine H-2 receptor antagonists (nizatidine, famotidine), antiparkinsonian and antiviral agents (amantadine), antidepressants (reboxetine, fluoxetine, fluvoxamine), and others [74, 75]. However, few randomized clinical trials exist that test these agents among overweight or obese patients with schizophrenia. Approaches include the prevention of excessive weight gain when starting an antipsychotic, or the loss of weight already gained after receiving an antipsychotic for some time. Most of the studies enrolled small numbers of subjects and have mainly focused on ameliorating the weight gain observed with olanzapine. The randomized double-blind studies of these adjunctive agents [76–101] are summarized in table 4. Results are generally inconsistent. Many interventions as tested do not show a clinically significant benefit. Moreover, all adjunctive

Table 4. Double-blind, randomized, clinical trials for non-FDA-approved adjunctive pharmacological interventions for weight gain among patients with schizophrenia

Author	Study medication (dose or dose range, with reported frequency)	Antipsychotic received (and other qualifications)	Study length weeks	n	Helpful?	Weight change observed in intervention group (vs. control group)
Graham [77]	amantadine (up to 300 mg/day)	olanzapine (and weight gain of at least 5 lb)	12	21	yes	BMI –0.07 (vs. +1.24)
Deberdt [78]	amantadine (100-300 mg/day)	olanzapine (and weight gain of at least 5%)	16 (24)	125	maybe	–0.19 kg (vs. +1.28 kg) but results at 24 weeks were not statistically significantly different
Cavazzoni [79]	nizatidine (150 mg b.i.d. or 300 mg b.i.d.)	olanzapine (newly started)	16	175	no	difference was not statistically significant at 16 weeks
Atmaca [80]	nizatidine (150 mg b.i.d.)	olanzapine (and weight gain in the range of 2.6–10.8 kg)	8	35	yes	–4.5 kg (vs. +2.3 kg)
Atmaca [81]	nizatidine (150 mg b.i.d.)	quetiapine (and weight gain in the range of 2.3–7.2 kg)	8	28	no	difference was not statistically significant
Assunção [82]	nizatidine (300 mg BID)	olanzapine (and weight gain of at least 5% from baseline)	12	54	no	difference was not statistically significant
Poyurovsky [83]	famotidine (40 mg/day)	olanzapine (first-episode patients)	6	14	no	difference was not statistically significant
Baptista [76]	metformin (850 mg/day – 850 mg b.i.d.) with sibutramine (10 mg/ day – 10 mg b.i.d.)	olanzapine	12	28	no	difference was not statistically significant
Wu [88]	metformin (250 mg t.i.d.)	olanzapine (drug-naïve first-episode patients)	12	40	yes	+1.9 kg (vs. +6.87 kg); number experiencing weight gain greater than 7% was 16.7% (vs. 63.2%)
Wu [89]	metformin (250 mg t.i.d.) and/or lifestyle intervention	clozapine, olanzapine, risperidone, sulpiride (and weight gain of more than 10%)	12	128	yes	lifestyle-plus-metformin group BMI –1.8 (vs. metformin-alone group –1.2 vs. lifestyle-plus-placebo group –0.5 vs. placebo group +1.2)

Table 4. Continued

Author	Study medication (dose or dose range, with reported frequency)	Antipsychotic received (and other qualifications)	Study length weeks	n	Helpful?	Weight change observed in intervention group (vs. control group)
Klein [90]	metformin (500 mg/day – 850 mg b.i.d.)	olanzapine, risperidone, or quetiapine (and weight gain of more than 10%; children ages 10-17 years)	16	39	yes	stable weight (vs. +0.31 kg/week)
Baptista [91]	metformin (850–1,700 mg/day)	olanzapine	14	40	no	difference was not statistically significant
Baptista [92]	metformin (850–2,550 mg/day)	olanzapine	12	80	no	difference was not statistically significant
Ko [84]	topiramate (50 mg b.i.d. or 100 mg b.i.d.)	risperidone, olanzapine, quetiapine, or clozapine (and BMI of at least 25)	12	66	yes	–5.35 kg for topiramate 200 mg/day (vs. –1.68 kg for topiramate 100 mg/day vs. –0.3 kg for placebo)
Kim [85][a]	topiramate (50 mg b.i.d.)	olanzapine	12	60	yes	+2.66 kg (vs. +4.02 kg)
Nickel [86] Egger [87]	topiramate (250 mg/day)	olanzapine (only women who had gained at least 5 kg; psychosis or bipolar)	10	43	yes	–4.4 kg (vs. +1.2 kg); at the end of an open-label 18 month observation period, –9.4 kg (vs. +5.5 kg)
McElroy [72][a]	topiramate (25–600 mg/day) or sibutramine (5–15 mg/day)	various (bipolar patients, of which only 16 were receiving antipsychotics, and BMI of at least 30, or at least 27 kg/m^2 with concomitant obesity-related risk factors or diseases)	24	46	maybe	patients randomized either to sibutramine or topiramate lost comparable amounts of weight (4.1 and 2.8 kg, respectively)
Poyurovsky [98]	reboxetine (2 mg b.i.d.)	olanzapine (first-episode patients)	6	60	yes	+3.31 kg (vs. +4.91 kg); number experiencing weight gain greater than 7% was 19.4% (vs. 46.4%)

Table 4. Continued

Author	Study medication (dose or dose range, with reported frequency)	Antipsychotic received (and other qualifications)	Study length weeks	n	Helpful?	Weight change observed in intervention group (vs. control group)
Poyurovsky [97]	reboxetine (2 mg b.i.d.)	olanzapine (first-episode patients)	6	26	yes	+2.5 kg (vs. +5.5 kg); number experiencing weight gain greater than 7% was 20% (vs. 70%)
Poyurovsky [94]	fluoxetine (20 mg/day)	olanzapine (first-episode patients)	8	30	no	difference was not statistically significant
Bustillo [95]	fluoxetine (20–60 mg/day)	olanzapine (and gained at least 3% of weight)	16	30	no	+3 kg (vs. +1.7 kg)
Lu [96][a]	fluvoxamine (50 mg/day)	clozapine (250 mg/day or less or 600 mg/d or less)	12	68	maybe	+0.9 kg (vs. +3.2 kg)
Borovicka [93]	phenylpropanolamine (75 mg/day)	clozapine (and weight gain of more than 10%)	12	16	no	difference was not statistically significant
Goodall [99]	fenfluramine (15 mg b.i.d.)	depot fluphenazine, flupenthixol, or clopenthixol (and BMI of at least)	12	29	maybe	rate of weight loss was significantly greater in those taking D-fenfluramine among the completers
Modell [100]	dextroamphetamine (5 mg/day)	thioridazine, chlorpromazine	8	20	no	+0.11 kg/week (vs. +0.01 kg/week)
Ding [101]	ling gui zhu gan tang mixture	clozapine, chlorpromazine, perphenazine, risperidone, sulpiride, trifluoperazine (and body weight exceeding 20% of standard)	8	100	yes	–4.5 kg (vs. +5.0 kg)

[a] Although randomized, this study was not double-blind.

medications may pose a tolerability problem for some patients, for example topiramate may be associated with cognitive dulling which can complicate the successful treatment of a patient with schizophrenia who may already be experiencing cognitive dysfunction [102]. Adjunctive reboxetine may be useful in preventing weight gain in first-episode patients [97, 98], but is currently not available in the USA. There are some non-Western treatments that may be helpful [101]. The adjunctive agent that holds the most promise, at least for persons early on in their illness, is adjunctive metformin [88–92].

Bariatric Surgery

There are no published controlled trials for the use of surgical interventions for the treatment of obesity for patients with schizophrenia. However, there is a report of a case series of 5 patients with schizophrenia and morbid obesity and a comparison was made with 165 nonpsychotic patients who also underwent bariatric surgery during a 1-year period [103]. The median BMI was 54 and all had obesity-related comorbidities, and all patients had been previously treated unsuccessfully with conservative methods of weight reduction. Median percent excess weight loss at 6 months was comparable to that achieved in the control group: excess weight loss was 39.5% in the patients with schizophrenia versus 46.9% in the controls (difference not statistically significant). In severely obese individuals with schizophrenia who have failed other attempts to address their disease, a careful individualized risk-to-benefit assessment for bariatric surgery should be considered. While having a history of a mental illness should not prevent people from getting bariatric surgery, evaluation of an individuals' preoperative psychiatric status may play an important role in maximizing successful postoperative outcomes [104].

Conclusions

Overweight and obese individuals with serious mental illnesses are at high risk for many medical problems, particularly cardiovascular morbidity and mortality. When added weight is concentrated viscerally, the expected result is insulin resistance and the eventual development of type 2 diabetes mellitus for those vulnerable individuals whose pancreas can no longer compensate by producing additional insulin.

The accumulation of excess body weight among patients with schizophrenia is multi-factorial, including unhealthy dietary choices, sedentary lifestyles and lack of access to appropriate food and physical activity sources, and perhaps a genetic or an intrinsic disease-state vulnerability for abdominal adiposity. Psychotropic medication, in particular the second-generation antipsychotics, have been associated with weight gain. These agents differ in their propensity for weight gain, with clozapine and olanzapine having the greatest likelihood of being associated with weight gain, and ziprasidone and aripiprazole the least. Switching from one agent to another, when clinically feasible, may help ameliorate weight gain. However, children, adolescents, and patients in their first episode of psychosis are at high risk for weight gain even with agents that are considered 'weight-neutral.' Monitoring weight is essential in individuals with mental illness receiving medication treatment, and early intervention to reduce weight or prevent further weight gain is crucial in order to avoid becoming overweight or obese.

Prevention of weight gain is indicated in any patient with a BMI of ≥25, and weight loss for any patient who has a BMI of ≥30 or a BMI of 25–29.9 and concomitant risk factors (such as hypertension, dyslipdemia, cardiovascular disease, diabetes, or sleep apnea [105]). Lifestyle and other nonpharmacological approaches show greater promise than using adjunctive medication treatments for weight loss, and the use of the latter requires nonpharmacological approaches to be in place in any event. The 'small steps approach' of setting modest nutritional and physical activity goals using accessible and realistic methods, is achievable during the routine care of individuals with serious mental illnesses.

References

1 Must A, Spadano J, Coakley EH, Field AE, Colditz G, Dietz WH: The disease burden associated with overweight and obesity. JAMA 1999;282:1523–1529.

2 Lois K, Young J, Kumar S: Obesity: eiphenomenon or cause of metabolic syndrome? Int J Clin Pract 2008;62:932–938.

3 Thakore JH, Mann JN, Vlahos I, Martin A, Reznek R: Increased visceral fat distribution in drug-naive and drug-free patients with schizophrenia. Int J Obes Relat Metab Disord 2002;26:137–141.

4 Citrome L, Volavka J: Atypical antipsychotics: revolutionary or incremental advance? Expert Rev Neurother 2002;2:69–88.

5 Weiden PJ, Mackell JA, McDonnell DD: Obesity as a risk factor for antipsychotic noncompliance. Schizophr Res 2004;66:51–57.

6 Bray GA: Evaluation of obesity. Postgrad Med 2003;114(6):19–38.

7 Citrome L: Metabolic syndrome and cardiovascular disease. J Psychopharmacol 2005;19(suppl):84–93.

8 Tan CE, Ma S, Wai D, Chew SK, Tai ES: Can we apply the National Cholesterol Education Program Adult Treatment Panel definition of the metabolic syndrome to Asians? Diabetes Care 2004;27:1182–1186.

9 Anuurad E, Shiwaku K, Nogi A, Kitajima K, Enkhmaa B, Shimono K, Yamane Y: The new BMI criteria for Asians by the regional office for the western pacific region of WHO are suitable for screening of overweight to prevent metabolic syndrome in elder Japanese workers. J Occup Health 2003;45:335–343.

10 Moyad MA: Fad diets and obesity. 1. Measuring weight in a clinical setting. Urol Nurs 2004;24:114–119.

11 James PT, Rigby N, Leach R, International Obesity Task Forc: The obesity epidemic, metabolic syndrome and future prevention strategies. Eur J Cardiovasc Prev Rehabil. 2004;11:3–8.

12 Silventoinen K, Sans S, Tolonen H, Monterde D, Kuulasmaa K, Kesteloot H, Tuomilehto J: Trends in obesity and energy supply in the WHO MONICA Project. Int J Obes Relat Metab Disord 2004;28:710–718.

13 Rennie KL, Jebb SA: Prevalence of obesity in Great Britain. Obes Rev 2005;6:11–12.

14 Ogden CL, Carroll MD, Curtin LR, McDowell MA, Tabak CJ, Flegal KM: Prevalence of overweight and obesity in the United States, 1999–2004. JAMA 2006; 295:1549–1555.

15 Allison DB, Fontaine KR, Heo M, Mentore JL, Cappelleri JC, Chandler LP, Weiden PJ, Cheskin LJ: The distribution of body mass index among individuals with and without schizophrenia. J Clin Psychiatry 1999;60:215–220.

16 McEvoy JP, Meyer JM, Goff DC, Nasrallah HA, Davis SM, Sullivan L, Meltzer HY, Hsiao J, Scott Stroup T, Lieberman JA: Prevalence of the metabolic syndrome in patients with schizophrenia: baseline results from the Clinical Antipsychotic Trials of Intervention Effectiveness (CATIE) schizophrenia trial and comparison with national estimates from NHANES III. Schizophr Res 2005; 80:19–32.

17 Rosenbaum M, Leibel RL, Hirsch J: Obesity. N Engl J Med 1997;337:396–407.

18 Menzel P, D'Aluisio F: Hungry Planet. Napa, Material World Books, 2005.

19 McCreadie RG, Kelly C, Connolly M, Williams S, Baxter G, Lean M, Paterson JR: Dietary improvement in people with schizophrenia: randomised controlled trial. Br J Psychiatry 2005;187:346–351.
20 Fava M, Judge R, Hoog SL, Nilsson ME, Koke SC: Fluoxetine versus sertraline and paroxetine in major depressive disorder: changes in weight with long-term treatment. J Clin Psychiatry 2000;61:863–867.
21 Vanina Y, Podolskaya A, Sedky K, Shahab H, Siddiqui A, Munshi F, Lippmann S: Body weight changes associated with psychopharmacology. Psychiatr Serv 2002;53:842–847.
22 Zimmermann U, Kraus T, Himmerich H, Schuld A, Pollmächer T: Epidemiology, implications and mechanisms underlying drug-induced weight gain in psychiatric patients. J Psychiatr Res 2003;37:193–220.
23 Matsui-Sakata A, Ohtani H, Sawada Y: Receptor occupancy-based analysis of the contributions of various receptors to antipsychotics-induced weight gain and diabetes mellitus. Drug Metab Pharmacokinet 2005;20:368–378.
24 Allison DB, Mentore JL, Heo M, Chandler LP, Cappelleri JC, Infante MC, Weiden PJ: Antipsychotic-induced weight gain: a comprehensive research synthesis. Am J Psychiatry 1999;156:1686–1696.
25 McIntyre RS, Trakas K, Lin D, Balshaw R, Hwang P, Robinson K, Eggleston A: Risk of weight gain associated with antipsychotic treatment: results from the Canadian National Outcomes Measurement Study in Schizophrenia. Can J Psychiatry 2003;48: 689–694.
26 Lieberman JA, Stroup TS, McEvoy JP, Swartz MS, Rosenheck RA, Perkins DO, Keefe RS, Davis SM, Davis CE, Lebowitz BD, Severe J, Hsiao JK, Clinical Antipsychotic Trials of Intervention Effectiveness (CATIE) Investigators: Effectiveness of antipsychotic drugs in patients with chronic schizophrenia. N Engl J Med 2005;353:1209–1223.
27 Citrome L, Stroup TS: Schizophrenia, Clinical Antipsychotic Trials of Intervention Effectiveness (CATIE) and number needed to treat: how can CATIE inform clinicians? Int J Clin Pract 2006;60: 933–940.
28 Citrome L: Compelling or irrelevant? Using number needed to treat can help decide. Acta Psychiatr Scand 2008;117:412–419.
29 Citrome L: The effectiveness criterion: balancing efficacy against the risk of weight gain. J Clin Psychiatry 2007;68(suppl 12):12–17.
30 Stroup TS, Lieberman JA, McEvoy JP, Swartz MS, Davis SM, Rosenheck RA, Perkins DO, Keefe RS, Davis CE, Severe J, Hsiao JK, CATIE Investigators: Effectiveness of olanzapine, quetiapine, risperidone, and ziprasidone in patients with chronic schizophrenia following discontinuation of a previous atypical antipsychotic. Am J Psychiatry 2006;163: 611–622.
31 Meyer JM, Pandina G, Bossie CA, Turkoz I, Greenspan A: Effects of switching from olanzapine to risperidone on the prevalence of the metabolic syndrome in overweight or obese patients with schizophrenia or schizoaffective disorder: analysis of a multicenter, rater-blinded, open-label study. Clin Ther 2005;27:1930–1941.
32 Weiden PJ, Daniel DG, Simpson G, Romano SJ: Improvement in indices of health status in outpatients with schizophrenia switched to ziprasidone. J Clin Psychopharmacol 2003;23:595–600.
33 Casey DE, Carson WH, Saha AR, Liebeskind A, Ali MW, Jody D, Ingenito GG, Aripiprazole Study Group: Switching patients to aripiprazole from other antipsychotic agents: a multicenter randomized study. Psychopharmacology (Berl) 2003;166: 391–399.
34 Kinon BJ, Kaiser CJ, Ahmed S, Rotelli MD, Kollack-Walker S: Association between early and rapid weight gain and change in weight over one year of olanzapine therapy in patients with schizophrenia and related disorders. J Clin Psychopharmacol 2005; 25:255–258.
35 Lipkovich I, Citrome L, Perlis R, Deberdt W, Houston JP, Ahl J, Hardy T: Early predictors of substantial weight gain in bipolar patients treated with olanzapine. J Clin Psychopharmacol 2006;26:316–320.
36 Kinon BJ, Basson BR, Gilmore JA, Tollefson GD: Long-term olanzapine treatment: weight change and weight-related health factors in schizophrenia. J Clin Psychiatry 2001;62:92–100.
37 Brecher M, Leong RW, Stening G, Osterling-Koskinen L, Jones AM: Quetiapine and long-term weight change: a comprehensive data review of patients with schizophrenia. J Clin Psychiatry 2007; 68:597–603.
38 Kinon BJ, Volavka J, Stauffer V, Edwards SE, Liu-Seifert H, Chen L, Adams DH, Lindemayer JP, McEvoy JP, Buckley PF, Lieberman JA, Meltzer HY, Eilson DR, Citrome L: Standard and higher dose of olanzapine in patients with schizophrenia or schizoaffective disorder: a randomized, double-blind, fixed dose study. J Clin Psychopharmacol 2008;28: 392–400.
39 Lane HY, Chang YC, Cheng YC, Liu GC, Lin XR, Chang WH: Effects of patient demographics, risperidone dosage, and clinical outcome on body weight in acutely exacerbated schizophrenia. J Clin Psychiatry 2003;64:316–320.
40 Arvanitis LA, Miller BG: Multiple fixed doses of 'Seroquel' (quetiapine) in patients with acute exacerbation of schizophrenia: a comparison with haloperidol and placebo: the Seroquel Trial 13 Study Group. Biol Psychiatry 1997;42:233–246.

41 Correll CU: Weight gain and metabolic effects of mood stabilizers and antipsychotics in pediatric bipolar disorder: a systematic review and pooled analysis of short-term trials. J Am Acad Child Adolesc Psychiatry 2007;46:687–700.
42 Strassnig M, Miewald J, Keshavan M, Ganguli R: Weight gain in newly diagnosed first-episode psychosis patients and healthy comparisons: one-year analysis. Schizophr Res 2007;93:90–98.
43 McEvoy JP, Lieberman JA, Perkins DO, Hamer RM, Gu H, Lazarus A, Sweitzer D, Olexy C, Weiden P, Strakowski SD: Efficacy and tolerability of olanzapine, quetiapine, and risperidone in the treatment of early psychosis: a randomized, double-blind 52-week comparison. Am J Psychiatry 2007;164: 1050–1060.
44 Kahn RS, Fleischhacker WW, Boter H, Davidson M, Vergouwe Y, Keet IP, Gheorghe MD, Rybakowski JK, Galderisi S, Libiger J, Hummer M, Dollfus S, López-Ibor JJ, Hranov LG, Gaebel W, Peuskens J, Lindefors N, Riecher-Rössler A, Grobbee DE, EUFEST Study Group: Effectiveness of antipsychotic drugs in first-episode schizophrenia and schizophreniform disorder: an open randomised clinical trial. Lancet 2008;371:1085–1097.
45 American Diabetes Association, American Psychiatric Association, American Association of Clinical Endocrinologists, North American Association for the Study of Obesity: Consensus Development Conference on Antipsychotic Drugs and Obesity and Diabetes. Diabetes Care 2004;27: 596–601.
46 Harmatz MG, Lapuc P: Behavior modification of overeating in a psychiatric population. J Consult Clin Psychol 1968;32:583–587.
47 Wu MK, Wang CK, Bai YM, Huang CY, Lee SD: Outcomes of obese, clozapine-treated inpatients with schizophrenia placed on a six-month diet and physical activity program. Psychiatr Serv 2007;58: 544–550.
48 Mauri M, Simoncini M, Castrogiovanni S, Iovieno N, Cecconi D, Dell'Agnello G, Quadrigli M, Rossi A, Donda P, Fagiolini A, Cassano GB: A psychoeducational program for weight loss in patients who have experienced weight gain during antipsychotic treatment with olanzapine. Pharmacopsychiatry 2008;41: 17–23.
49 Alvarez-Jiménez M, González-Blanch C, Vázquez-Barquero JL, Pérez-Iglesias R, Martínez-García O, Pérez-Pardal T, Ramírez-Bonilla ML, Crespo-Facorro B: Attenuation of antipsychotic-induced weight gain with early behavioral intervention in drug-naive first-episode psychosis patients: A randomized controlled trial. J Clin Psychiatry 2006;67: 1253–1260.
50 Littrell KH, Hilligoss NM, Kirshner CD, Petty RG, Johnson CG: The effects of an educational intervention on antipsychotic-induced weight gain. J Nurs Scholarsh 2003;35:237–241.
51 Evans S, Newton R, Higgins S: Nutritional intervention to prevent weight gain in patients commenced on olanzapine: a randomized controlled trial. Aust N Z J Psychiatry 2005;39:479–486.
52 Vreeland B, Minsky S, Menza M, Rigassio Radler D, Roemheld-Hamm B, Stern R: A program for managing weight gain associated with atypical antipsychotics. Psychiatr Serv 2003;54:1155–1157.
53 Menza M, Vreeland B, Minsky S, Gara M, Radler DR, Sakowitz M: Managing atypical antipsychotic-associated weight gain: 12-month data on a multimodal weight control program. J Clin Psychiatry 2004;65:471–477.
54 Ball MP, Coons VB, Buchanan RW: A program for treating olanzapine-related weight gain. Psychiatr Serv 2001;52:967–969.
55 Brar JS, Ganguli R, Pandina G, Turkoz I, Berry S, Mahmoud R: Effects of behavioral therapy on weight loss in overweight and obese patients with schizophrenia or schizoaffective disorder. J Clin Psychiatry 2005;66:205–212.
56 Kwon JS, Choi JS, Bahk WM, Yoon Kim C, Hyung Kim C, Chul Shin Y, Park BJ, Geun Oh C: Weight management program for treatment-emergent weight gain in olanzapine-treated patients with schizophrenia or schizoaffective disorder: a 12-week randomized controlled clinical trial. J Clin Psychiatry 2006;67:547–553.
57 Weber M, Wyne K: A cognitive/behavioral group intervention for weight loss in patients treated with atypical antipsychotics. Schizophr Res 2006;83:95–101.
58 Khazaal Y, Fresard E, Rabia S, Chatton A, Rothen S, Pomini V, Grasset F, Borgeat F, Zullino D: Cognitive behavioural therapy for weight gain associated with antipsychotic drugs. Schizophr Res 2007;91:169–177.
59 Brown S, Chan K: A randomized controlled trial of a brief health promotion intervention in a population with serious mental illness. J Ment Health 2006;15:543–549.
60 McKibbin CL, Patterson TL, Norman G, Patrick K, Jin H, Roesch S, Mudaliar S, Barrio C, O'Hanlon K, Griver K, Sirkin A, Jeste DV: A lifestyle intervention for older schizophrenia patients with diabetes mellitus: a randomized controlled trial. Schizophr Res 2006;86:36–44.
61 Rotatori AF, Fox R, Wicks A: Weight loss with psychiatric residents in a behavioral self control program. Psychol Rep 1980;46:483–486.
62 National Heart Lung and Blood Institute, North American Association for the Study of Obesity: The Practical Guide: Identification, Evaluation, and Treatment of Overweight and Obesity in Adults. Bethesda, National Institutes of Health, 2000.
63 Tsai AG, Wadden TA, Womble LG, Byrne KJ: Commercial and self-help programs for weight control. Psychiatr Clin North Am 2005;28:171–192.

64 Dansinger ML, Gleason JA, Griffith JL, Selker HP, Schaefer EJ: Comparison of the Atkins, Ornish, Weight Watchers, and Zone diets for weight loss and heart disease risk reduction: a randomized trial. JAMA 2005;293:43–53.

65 Hoffmann VP, Ahl J, Meyers A, Schuh L, Shults KS, Collins DM, Jensen L: Wellness intervention for patients with serious and persistent mental illness. J Clin Psychiatry 2005;66:1576–1579.

66 Vreeland B, Toto AM, Sakowitz M: Solutions for Wellness, ed 3. Indianapolis, Eli Lilly, 2008.

67 Hill JO, Wyatt HR: Small changes: a big idea for addressing obesity. Obesity Mgmt 2006;2:227–231.

68 Joffe G, Takala P, Tchoukhine E, Hakko H, Raidma M, Putkonen H, Eronen M, Räsänen P: Orlistat in clozapine- or olanzapine-treated patients with overweight or obesity: A 16-week randomized, double-blind, placebo-controlled trial. J Clin Psychiatry 2008;69:706–711.

69 Hilger E, Quiner S, Ginzel I, Walter H, Saria L, Barnas C: The effect of orlistat on plasma levels of psychotropic drugs in patients with long-term psychopharmacotherapy. J Clin Psychopharmacol 2002; 22:68–70.

70 Henderson DC, Copeland PM, Daley TB, Borba CP, Cather C, Nguyen DD, Louie PM, Evins AE, Freudenreich O, Hayden D, Goff DC: A double-blind, placebo-controlled trial of sibutramine for olanzapine-associated weight gain. Am J Psychiatry 2005;162:954–962.

71 Henderson DC, Fan X, Copeland PM, Borba CP, Daley TB, Nguyen DD, Zhang H, Hayden D, Freudenreich O, Cather C, Evins AE, Goff DC: A double-blind, placebo-controlled trial of sibutramine for clozapine-associated weight gain. Acta Psychiatr Scand 2007;115:101–105.

72 McElroy SL, Frye MA, Altshuler LL, Suppes T, Hellemann G, Black D, Mintz J, Kupka R, Nolen W, Leverich GS, Denicoff KD, Post RM, Keck PE Jr: A 24-week, randomized, controlled trial of adjunctive sibutramine versus topiramate in the treatment of weight gain in overweight or obese patients with bipolar disorders. Bipolar Disord 2007;9:426–434.

73 Christensen R, Kristensen PK, Bartels EM, Bliddal H, Astrup A: Efficacy and safety of the weight-loss drug rimonabant: a meta-analysis of randomised trials. Lancet 2007;370:1706–1713.

74 Faulkner G, Cohn T, Remington G: Interventions to reduce weight gain in schizophrenia. Schizophr Bull 2007;33:654–656.

75 Faulkner G, Cohn T, Remington G: Interventions to reduce weight gain in schizophrenia. Cochrane Database Syst Rev 2007;1:CD005148.

76 Baptista T, Uzcátegui E, Rangel N, El Fakih Y, Galeazzi T, Beaulieu S, de Baptista EA: Metformin plus sibutramine for olanzapine-associated weight gain and metabolic dysfunction in schizophrenia: a 12-week double-blind, placebo-controlled pilot study. Psychiatry Res 2008;159:250–253.

77 Graham KA, Gu H, Lieberman JA, Harp JB, Perkins DO: Double-blind, placebo-controlled investigation of amantadine for weight loss in subjects who gained weight with olanzapine. Am J Psychiatry 2005;162:1744–1746.

78 Deberdt W, Winokur A, Cavazzoni PA, Trzaskoma QN, Carlson CD, Bymaster FP, Wiener K, Floris M, Breier A: Amantadine for weight gain associated with olanzapine treatment. Eur Neuropsychopharmacol 2005;15:13–21.

79 Cavazzoni P, Tanaka Y, Roychowdhury SM, Breier A, Allison DB: Nizatidine for prevention of weight gain with olanzapine: a double-blind placebo-controlled trial. Eur Neuropsychopharmacol 2003;13: 81–85.

80 Atmaca M, Kuloglu M, Tezcan E, Ustundag B: Nizatidine treatment and its relationship with leptin levels in patients with olanzapine-induced weight gain. Hum Psychopharmacol 2003;18:457–461.

81 Atmaca M, Kuloglu M, Tezcan E, Ustundag B, Kilic N: Nizatidine for the treatment of patients with quetiapine-induced weight gain. Hum Psychopharmacol 2004;19:37–40.

82 Assunção SS, Ruschel SI, Rosa Lde C, Campos JA, Alves MJ, Bracco OL, de Lima MS: Weight gain management in patients with schizophrenia during treatment with olanzapine in association with nizatidine. Rev Bras Psiquiatr 2006 28:270–276.

83 Poyurovsky M, Tal V, Maayan R, Gil-Ad I, Fuchs C, Weizman A: The effect of famotidine addition on olanzapine-induced weight gain in first-episode schizophrenia patients: a double-blind placebo-controlled pilot study. Eur Neuropsychopharmacol 2004;14:332–336.

84 Ko YH, Joe SH, Jung IK, Kim SH: Topiramate as an adjuvant treatment with atypical antipsychotics in schizophrenic patients experiencing weight gain. Clin Neuropharmacol 2005;28:169–175.

85 Kim JH, Yim SJ, Nam JH: A 12-week, randomized, open-label, parallel-group trial of topiramate in limiting weight gain during olanzapine treatment in patients with schizophrenia. Schizoph Res 2006;82:115–117.

86 Nickel MK, Nickel C, Muehlbacher M, Leiberich PK, Kaplan P, Lahmann C, Tritt K, Krawczyk J, Kettler C, Egger C, Rother WK, Loew TH: Influence of topiramate on olanzapine-related adiposity in women: a random, double-blind, placebo-controlled study. J Clin Psychopharmacol 2005;25:211–217.

87 Egger C, Muehlbacher M, Schatz M, Nickel M: Influence of topiramate on olanzapine-related weight gain in women: an 18-month follow-up observation. J Clin Psychopharmacol 2007;27:475–478.
88 Wu RR, Zhao JP, Guo XF, He YQ, Fang MS, Guo WB, Chen JD, Li LH: Metformin addition attenuates olanzapine-induced weight gain in drug-naive first-episode schizophrenia patients: a double-blind, placebo-controlled study. Am J Psychiatry 2008; 165:352–358.
89 Wu RR, Zhao JP, Jin H, Shao P, Fang MS, Guo XF, He YQ, Liu YJ, Chen JD, Li LH: Lifestyle intervention and metformin for treatment of antipsychotic-induced weight gain: a randomized controlled trial. JAMA 2008;299:185–193.
90 Klein DJ, Cottingham EM, Sorter M, Barton BA, Morrison JA: A randomized, double-blind, placebo-controlled trial of metformin treatment of weight gain associated with initiation of atypical antipsychotic therapy in children and adolescents. Am J Psychiatry 2006;163:2072–2079.
91 Baptista T, Martínez J, Lacruz A, Rangel N, Beaulieu S, Serrano A, Arapé Y, Martinez M, de Mendoza S, Teneud L, Hernández L: Metformin for prevention of weight gain and insulin resistance with olanzapine: a double-blind placebo-controlled trial. Can J Psychiatry 2006;51:192–196.
92 Baptista T, Rangel N, Fernández V, Carrizo E, El Fakih Y, Uzcátegui E, Galeazzi T, Gutiérrez MA, Servigna M, Dávila A, Uzcátegui M, Serrano A, Connell L, Beaulieu S, de Baptista EA: Metformin as an adjunctive treatment to control body weight and metabolic dysfunction during olanzapine administration: a multicentric, double-blind, placebo-controlled trial. Schizophr Res 2007;93:99–108.
93 Borovicka MC, Fuller MA, Konicki PE, White JC, Steele VM, Jaskiw GE: Phenylpropanolamine appears not to promote weight loss in patients with schizophrenia who have gained weight during clozapine treatment. J Clin Psychiatry 2002;63:345–348.
94 Poyurovsky M, Pashinian A, Gil-Ad I, Maayan R, Schneidman M, Fuchs C, Weizman A: Olanzapine-induced weight gain in patients with first-episode schizophrenia: a double-blind, placebo-controlled study of fluoxetine addition. Am J Psychiatry 2002;159:1058–1060.
95 Bustillo JR, Lauriello J, Parker K, Hammond R, Rowland L, Bogenschutz M, Keith S: Treatment of weight gain with fluoxetine in olanzapine-treated schizophrenic outpatients. Neuropsychopharmacology 2003;28:527–529.
96 Lu ML, Lane HY, Lin SK, Chen KP, Chang WH: Adjunctive fluvoxamine inhibits clozapine-related weight gain and metabolic disturbances. J Clin Psychiatry 2004;65:766–771.
97 Poyurovsky M, Isaacs I, Fuchs C, Schneidman M, Faragian S, Weizman R, Weizman A: Attenuation of olanzapine-induced weight gain with reboxetine in patients with schizophrenia: a double-blind, placebo-controlled study. Am J Psychiatry 2003;160:297–302.
98 Poyurovsky M, Fuchs C, Pashinian A, Levi A, Faragian S, Maayan R, Gil-Ad I: Attenuating effect of reboxetine on appetite and weight gain in olanzapine-treated schizophrenia patients: a double-blind placebo-controlled study. Psychopharmacology (Berl) 2007;192:441–448.
99 Goodall E, Oxtoby C, Richards R, Watkinson G, Brown D, Silverstone T: A clinical trial of the efficacy and acceptability of D-fenfluramine in the treatment of neuroleptic-induced obesity. Br J Psychiatry 1988;153:208–213.
100 Modell W, Hussar AE: Failure of dextroamphetamine sulfate to influence eating and sleeping patterns in obese schizophrenic patients: clinical and pharmacological significance. JAMA 1965;193:95–98.
101 Ding G, Yu G, Zhang J, Liang S, Liu L, Huang P, Chen H, Xiao A, Li X, Cai Y: The therapeutic effects of ling gui zhu gan tang mixture in 50 psychotic patients with obesity induced by the psychoactive drugs. J Tradit Chin Med 2005;25:25–28.
102 Duggal HS: Psychotic symptoms associated with topiramate: cognitive side effects or worsening of psychosis? J Clin Psychiatry 2004;65:1145.
103 Hamoui N, Kingsbury S, Anthone GJ, Crookes PF: Surgical treatment of morbid obesity in schizophrenic patients. Obes Surg 2004;14:349–352.
104 Sarwer DB, Cohn NI, Gibbons LM, Magee L, Crerand CE, Raper SE, Rosato EF, Williams NN, Wadden TA: Psychiatric diagnoses and psychiatric treatment among bariatric surgery candidates. Obes Surg 2004;14:1148–1156.
105 Clinical guidelines on the identification, evaluation, and treatment of overweight and obesity in adults: executive summary. Expert panel on the identification, evaluation, and treatment of overweight in adults. Am J Clin Nutr 1998;68:899–917.

Leslie Citrome, MD, MPH
Nathan S. Kline Institute for Psychiatric Research
140 Old Orangeburg Road
Orangeburg, NY 10962 (USA)
Tel. +1 845 398 5595, Fax +1 845 398 5483, E-Mail citrome@nki.rfmh.org

Thakore J, Leonard BE (eds): Metabolic Effects of Psychotropic Drugs.
Mod Trends Pharmacopsychiatry. Basel, Karger, 2009, vol 26, pp 47–65

Glucose Abnormalities in Schizophrenia, Bipolar and Major Depressive Disorders

Chris Bushe

Eli Lilly and Company, Basingstoke, UK

Abstract

Glucose abnormalities have been recognised to be important parameters that may predict many adverse cardiovascular outcomes in the general population. Their description is complex and more so in patients suffering from mental disorders where the more formal measurements of fasting data become more difficult to obtain routinely. Despite this, there is clarity that abnormal glucose parameters may be found in at least 30% patients with severe forms of mental illness. This chapter aims to describe the available literature and attempt to better understand the plethora of data relating to glucose that derives from patients suffering from chronic mental disorders such as schizophrenia and mood disorders.

Glucose abnormalities have been recognised to be important parameters that may predict many adverse cardiovascular outcomes in the general population. Their description is complex and more so in patients suffering from mental disorders where the more formal measurements of fasting data become more difficult to obtain routinely. Despite this, there is clarity that abnormal glucose parameters may be found in at least 30% patients with severe forms of mental illness [1].

This chapter aims to describe the available literature and attempt to better understand the plethora of data relating to glucose that derives from patients suffering from chronic mental disorders such as schizophrenia and mood disorders. Where glucose abnormalities (diabetes and pre-diabetes) fit into the metabolic syndrome and indeed the validity of the metabolic syndrome, using current definitions in predicting adverse outcomes does not fall into the remit of this chapter nor do other forms of psychotic disorders.

Diabetes and Pre-Diabetes in the General Population

Diabetes (DM) type 2 is highly prevalent worldwide in 2008 and will have increasing prevalence through until at least 2025 coincident with a global obesity epidemic [2].

Diabetes type 1 is a very different disorder that is predominantly genetically inherited and in which obesity is not an important risk factor. Worldwide there are substantial regional variations with Africa having the lowest prevalence. In Europe, prevalence will increase from around 6% in 2008 to 8% in 2025 in the 20–79 age group and in some regions will increase to over 10% [2]. The worldwide prevalence of DM was 5.1% in 2003 and will rise to 6.3% by 2005. In the UK it is estimated that by 2010 DM will be diagnosed in 7% of men and 5% of women [3]. In addition, impaired glucose tolerance (IGT) will rise from 8.2% in 2003 to 9% in 2005. The sheer relevance of these data is encapsulated in the single statistic that in 2007 3.8 million deaths will be due to DM globally [4]. Complications of DM are of concern on many levels in that peripheral vascular disease (amputation risk is increased by 15–40 times compared with the general population), retinopathy and cardiovascular disease are mostly also irreversible once initiated, although there are some modern management techniques that benefit patients [4]. Many subjects with glucose abnormalities remain undiagnosed which may increase these figures further and within this group there may be very specific populations, including the family members of patients with severe mental illness who could be targeting for screening. Using data from NHANES, the prevalence of DM and impaired fasting glycaemia (IFG) in adults >20 years of age was 5.9% and 6.1%, respectively, in 2000 (but DM increasing to 15% in >60 years), which increased to 8.3% when adding undiagnosed DM [5].

Prevalence of Glucose Abnormalities in Schizophrenia

Diabetes

It has been established for over 100 years that glucose abnormalities are more frequent in mentally ill subjects [6] and without doubt predate the emergence of antipsychotic treatments. The precise prevalence and incidence rates are only starting to be described and are in part dependent on the cohort evaluated and the year of study. Screening for glucose abnormalities has increased since 2000 and data prior to then are less complicated in their interpretation. A lifetime DM prevalence of 15% was reported from the Schizophrenia Patient Outcomes Research Team (PORT) in the USA in data collected dirung the mid-1990s prior to atypicals [7]. The data were stringently collected with subjects being paid for their time spent in interview. In 2002, a prevalence rate of 18% in an outpatient cohort was noteworthy for the clear findings that the prevalence increased with age, as in the general population, with the highest prevalence of >25% in the 60- to 69-year cohort [8]. In some cohort studies, prevalence rates can be compared with those in the general population at that time. Prevalence rates of 15.8% in Italy, in a schizophrenia cohort admitted to a long-term care facility, vastly exceeded the then current rates of 2–3% in the Italian general population [9]. There can be little doubt that not all patients were screened and screening bias needs to be factored in. For example, younger subjects may be more likely to be admitted and hence receive routine glucose tests. Prevalence in certain ethic groups may also be variable. Subramamiam et al. [10] reported on an inpatient cohort in Singapore where chart review found the DM prevalence rate to be 4.9% in a large cohort receiving typicals. Following an oral glucose tolerance test (OGTT), however, the overall prevalence rose to 21% emphasising the value of OGTT as a diagnostic tool. In the 50- to 59-year-old cohort, the prevalence was 50%. Screening bias, however, needs to be factored into any naturalistic data set. Data from the UK Maudsley and other local London trusts derived in 2002–2003 found that only 41% of inpatients had some form of glucose testing on case notes review [11, 12]. The actual prevalence rate for glycaemic abnormalities was more accurately determined as 15.6% (39 of 250 tested subjects) as opposed to a case notes review prevalence of 6.4% (39 of 606 subjects) of whom the vast majority had DM (n = 37) and only 2 patients had IFG. There were no reported cases of IGT strongly implying that this test had not been applied frequently. The very low prevalence of any form of pre-diabetic abnormality might suggest that abnormal glucose levels outside of diagnostic diabetic levels had not been considered relevant and not recorded. At that time, there may have been a lower awareness of the prognostic value and morbidity of pre-diabetes.

Data from USA in a chronic inpatient cohort of over 13,000 subjects with schizophrenia finds a prevalence of 11% [13]. These prevalence rates need to be contextualised with what is happening worldwide as, in the USA, the age-adjusted prevalence of obesity (BMI >30) in adults increased from 22.9% in 1988–1994 to 30.5% in 1999–2000 [14], and the age-adjusted prevalence of diagnosed diabetes in adults increased from 5.1% in 1997 to 6.5% in 2002 [5].

A lot of prevalence data are complex to interpret. A recent cross-sectional study of 210 subjects, despite reporting a prevalence for DM of only 4.8%, excluded subjects undergoing treatment for DM and the latter numbers are not often reported. When the additional 5.2% with IFG (>6.1 mmol/l) are included, the interpretation of these data might be that 10% had 'hidden' glucose abnormalities [15]. To calculate the true DM prevalence, it would be necessary to also know how many excluded subjects had current diagnoses of DM or pre-diabetes.

Over the last 5 years, data have begun to emerge on the incidence of DM in schizophrenia cohorts. These data are also complex to interpret as the incidence and prevalence of DM in the general population is rising. The question to focus on is whether the incidence rate of DM is rising faster in subjects with serious mental illness (SMI) than in the general population. This is not a question that can be answered at the present as screening bias in both populations remains both a caveat and a confounder. Some evidence that the incidence rate of DM is rising to a greater extent in the SMI population than in the general population derives from a large USA cohort study of inpatients with schizophrenia and bipolar disorder. In this cohort, the prevalence of diabetes increased from 6.9% in 1997 to 14.5% in 2004 [16] with associated increases in incidence rates of diabetes from 0.9% in 1997 to 1.8% in 2004. During the same period, the incidence of diabetes rose from 0.51 to 0.72% in the USA general population [17], and the age-adjusted prevalence of diabetes in adults increased from 5.1% in 1997 to 6.5% in 2002 [5]. Traditionally, in schizophrenia the lowest DM rates are measured in the age group 18–44 years [8]. In 2003, in the USA cohort the DM prevalence of 10.0% contrasts with 2.3% for the corresponding age cohort in the general population [16].

In a naturalistic Belgian cohort (n = 183), a 3-month incident rate of 4.4% (n = 8) for DM was reported using OGTT [18]; however, when screening the original cohort (n = 220), 5.5% had previously been diagnosed with DM. In the DM incident cohort 5 of the 8 subjects had forms of pre-diabetes at the study outset. These data are not dissimilar to other reported incidence rates. The same group have reported an annual incidence rate of 4.2% in an identically screened stable schizophrenia population [19], and other annual incidence rates of 3.2–3.6% [20] and 4.4% [21] in subjects newly commenced on antipsychotics have also been reported. Incidence rates are higher (4.7 and 6.9%) and more difficult to interpret from diagnostically mixed samples [22, 23]. In a large USA inpatient sample of chronic subjects, the annual incident rates during 2000–2002 were lower, i.e. 1.25–1.5%. This may reflect better previous screening [13].

The Belgian group under De Hert has produced some interesting naturalistic data from a consecutive prospective cohort of 415 schizophrenia subjects [24]. They report that the difference in DM prevalence between schizophrenia subjects and a control population increases with increasing age being 1.6% in the 15- to 25-year cohort and 19.2% in the 55- to 65-year cohort. Using OGTT, they identified more DM cases than by fasting glycaemia (FG) alone which would have identified only 46.2% of DM cases. In comparing cohorts, they divided subjects into cohorts <1.5, <10 s, 10–20 and >20 years. The prevalence of DM increased from 3% in the early phase cohort to 16.5% in the chronic cohort and similarly the prevalence of FG >5.6 mmol/l (the inclusion criteria for metabolic syndrome IDF) was found to increase from 8 to 40.5%.

Pre-Diabetes

Although usage of this term may be technically inaccurate (as diabetes is not an inevitable outcome), it is useful to capture under a single metric the numbers of patients who cannot be diagnosed as DM but who have abnormal glucose values to some extent. Fasting glucose cannot always be obtained pragmatically in SMI patients both for psychiatric and logistical reasons. Many patients are unable to successfully fast perhaps due to failure to understand the precise and exact nature of the fast needed. In the UK, this has been acknowledged in two consensus group reports in 2004 and 2005 [25, 26]. In addition, although the ADA clearly state that an OGTT is an important diagnostic tool to diagnose all forms of glucose abnormality they also recognise the impracticality of general use. As a consequence, many current glucose measurements undertaken outside of a formal randomised control trial (RCT) are non-fasting and the sensitivity/specificity of a single glucose test may differ little between fasting and non-fasting [27]. Non-fasting also confers the benefit of no risk of overestimation of an abnormality. Pre-diabetes thus captures abnormal non-fasting levels, IGT and IFT as well as cases where repeat measurements are needed to confirm DM.

Data are relatively recent on the prevalence and incidence of pre-diabetes. The highest reported prevalence is 30–31% IGT [10, 28]. These data derive from a prospective cross-sectional studies and revealed large amounts of undiagnosed hyperglycaemia as almost all these patients were previously considered to be euglycaemic. The Sernyak study provided further insight into difficulties of obtaining fasting glucose samples. In a total of 647 outpatients receiving antipsychotics, an attempt was made to obtain a fasting sample. However, only 23.6% of the samples were fasting and 76.4% were random. Despite excluding all known diabetics 30.1% of the fasting samples had abnormally elevated glucose (24.8% fasting plasma glucose (FPG) 5.6–6.9 mmol/l; 5.2% (n = 8) FPG >7.0 mmol/l). In contrast, case-note reviews have reported prevalence rates as low as almost zero [11], implying that there may have been a failure to document abnormal glucose levels failing to reach a diabetogenic threshold. Psychiatrists in the UK may have been unaware of the prognostic importance of a pre-diabetic diagnosis. In one of a series of naturalistic data sets (n = 183) from Belgium [18] using OGTT, pre-diabetic abnormalities were reported in 16%. Following 3 months of antipsychotic treatments pre-diabetic abnormalities had regressed in 40% of the cases (n = 12) and had developed newly in 29 cases, giving a pre-diabetes prevalence at 3 months of 26%, emphasising the value of screening using OGTT where feasible (although usually impractical in SMI patients) as opposed to fasting samples.

Treatment-naïve cohorts have also suggested an elevated rate of glucose abnormalities compared to controls with Ryan et al. [29] reporting a 15% prevalence of IFG with no DM cases.

Mood Disorder

There is a general perception that glucose abnormalities in bipolar disorder are not dissimilar to schizophrenia. The recent NICE guidelines for bipolar disorder emphasise the importance of glucose monitoring [30]. The problem is untangling bipolar disorders (all types) from treatment disorders and unipolar depression. Accordingly, definitive data on glucose metabolism is less defined with a complete absence of treatment-naïve data.

Bipolar Disorder and Glucose

Although there are fewer data than in schizophrenia there is an acceptance that glucose abnormalities are more frequent in bipolar subjects than in the general population and there is likely to be a similar prevalence to the schizophrenia population

[9, 31]. A chart review of inpatients reported 26% prevalence [32]. Recent data are also supportive that metabolic syndrome of which glucose often forms an important parameter is also more prevalent than in the general population with rates of 30–32% reported [33, 34].

Depression and Glucose

There has been awareness for many years that some connection exists between depression and diabetes. The increased usage of antipsychotics in treating major depression may complicate the analysis of the relationship between the disease and the onset of diabetes. A recent large USA chart review found that in a cohort of psychiatric inpatients receiving antipsychotics, the largest diagnostic group was major depressive disorder (27.6% of the sample) comparing with schizophrenia (13.8%) with 54.2% of these depressed subjects receiving antipsychotics [35]. Further data are needed to confirm if this finding might apply in all countries. An additional complexity is the diagnostic uncertainty between unipolar depression and various forms of bipolar disorder.

Pre-diabetes is often found in subjects with various depressive diagnoses considered to be euglycaemic when tested [28]; however, the first observation that depression is associated with diabetes was made in 1684 [36]. A recent review concluded that the point prevalence of depression in diabetes is 11% and that dependent on methodology prevalence may be as high as 28.5% [37, 38]. Meta-analysis found from 20 studies that odds of depression in a diabetic cohort were twice that of the non-diabetic cohort (OR = 2.0, 95% CI 1.8–2.2) [38] and no differences in depression prevalence between type 1 and type 2 DM could be determined. Importantly, depression is also associated with worsening of glycaemic control and remission with a reduction in glycosylated haemoglobin [39]. Cortisol was originally suggested as a putative pathophysiological mechanism; however, hyperglycaemia itself may worsen the depressive illness [40]. The precise relationship between depression, its treatment and glycaemia is complex to fathom out but when cohorts with major depressive disorder are followed the incidence of diabetes is higher than anticipated [37]. The reasons are unclear but may involve increased activity of the sympathoadrenal system, antidepressant medications, inactivity or other physical health changes mediated by the depressive illness. An algorithm has been proposed for management utilising essentially the common treatments but emphasising the importance of the comorbidity of these bidirectional illnesses [37].

Potential Pathophysiological Mechanisms for Glucose Elevation

Unravelling the relative qualitative and quantitative components to determine precise causation has proven complex and thus far remains unknown. From the general population, we know that type 2 diabetes may take up to 10 years from initial abnormality to elevated glucose. No clinical trial in modern-day psychiatry exceeds 3 years [41]. Thus, proposed mechanisms are speculative and include weight-gain associated increases in insulin resistance, a direct toxic drug effect on muscle or adipose tissue leading to insulin resistance, stimulation of hepatic glucose production and inhibition of insulin release through pancreatic toxicity. The quantitative role of abnormally elevated amounts of visceral fat [42, 43] present in treatment-naïve subjects (over three times greater than that in controls) and any other additional genetic predisposition to DM versus any treatment or lifestyle associated association is unknown.

Some recent data have led some to hypothesize that in SMI patients there may be a maximal threshold beyond which obesity may not impact greatly on insulin resistance [44]. Data from a 6-month randomised trial of schizophrenia subjects with baseline BMI 28–30 randomised to olanzapine or risperidone found no worsening or differences between the groups on parameters such as insulin sensitivity and disposition index (measure of pancreatic beta-cell functioning) using intravenous glucose tolerance testing. Treatment-emergent weight gain and small increases in visceral fat were observed in both treatment groups The hypothesis suggested was that these data were consistent with a non-linear relationship between obesity and insulin resistance.

There have been a number of other studies, albeit small cohorts that have evaluated a variety of antipsychotics in forms of testing such as hyperinsulinaemic euglycaemic clamps [45], comparison of visceral fat [42, 43], and intravenous glucose tolerance tests [46, 47]. Some studies were carried out in healthy subjects, some in schizophrenia subjects and importantly some were limited to non-obese subjects. The studies, however, have been cross-sectional and open to confounding. In studies in healthy subjects [45], a significant confounder exists that the schizophrenia metabolism is clearly very different from the healthy volunteer and results may differ in schizophrenia patients and prospective studies may be too short to be definitive in light of the above caveats. Furthermore, some studies have been restricted to male subjects only [45] with current data showing that there are important sex differences in the metabolic response to antipsychotic treatments [48].

Nevertheless, these data may be significant in at least suggesting trial designs that should begin to define the pathophysiological mechanisms involved and provide some comparative antipsychotic data. Sowell et al. [49] reported in 2002 that in a 3-arm study for 15–17 days (n = 48) comparing olanzapine, risperidone and placebo using a hyperglycaemic euglycaemic clamp, there were no significant between-group differences in insulin secretion. In a small study (n = 29), Sacher et al. [45] reported that in healthy subjects after 10 days there was a higher incidence of decreased insulin sensitivity and elevated insulin levels during treatment with olanzapine compared to ziprasidone, although baseline irregularities in the olanzapine cohort need to be considered. Using a different technique, an intravenous glucose tolerance test, Henderson's group reported data from two studies. In the first study, a cross-sectional study, subjects taking clozapine and olanzapine were found to have significant insulin resistance and impairment of glucose effectiveness when compared to risperidone [46], but with no significant differences in FPG or lipid parameters. The second study compared olanzapine, quetiapine and placebo [47] using the same technique and found that whereas there were significant differences compared to placebo on all parameters, there were no significant differences between patients treated with olanzapine and quetiapine on parameters of insulin sensitivity, insulin resistance, fasting insulin and glucose levels nor lipids. Glucose effectiveness was, however, lower in the olanzapine cohort ($p = 0.03$). There was an absence of significant change in pancreatic beta-cell function in olanzapine subjects. Finally, also using IVGT, one study reported that adiposity levels (BMI and waist circumference) were strongly related to insulin resistance [50].

Not all studies are in agreement, however. A 2-week randomised study in schizophrenia subjects randomised to olanzapine or risperidone found no differences in insulin sensitivity, insulin or glucose levels or glucose effectiveness. However, subjects taking olanzapine were found to have a decreased insulin secretory response to a hyperglycaemic challenge [51] a similar finding to a study in dogs treated with olanzapine which found impaired beta-cell compensation [52]. Other studies have shown contrasting results with no evidence that healthy subjects treated for 2 weeks with olanzapine or risperidone had any impairment of the acute insulin secretory response [53].

There are some data suggesting that subjects with schizophrenia may not be metabolically identical to control subjects with a recent study finding that insulin homeostasis was different in clozapine obese subjects compared to non-psychiatric obesity being significantly worse [54].

Currently available data do not clearly define the changes in glucose metabolism that may be observed in patients receiving longer-term treatment with antipsychotics. Ideally, future data should be derived from prospective, longer-term studies done in schizophrenia subjects and comparing commonly used atypical antipsychotics? Results of longer-term studies may differ from findings in short-term trials

Genetics and Glucose Abnormalities

There is consistency that in schizophrenia subjects a positive family history of DM is found significantly more often than in a control population [9, 55, 56]. Recent data report prevalence figures of 31 and 34% [18, 57]. These data are also consistent with data from USA in which family history of diabetes in the general population has a significant powerful, independent and graded association with diabetes [58]. There are clear ethnic and geographical variations in the prevalence of diabetes worldwide and data are perhaps best considered when comparative data in that country are available. In 2006, the prevalence of type 2 DM in Barcelona was 8% [59]. In 2008, in 34 treatment-naïve subjects with non-affective forms of psychosis, a positive history of DM in either parent (27%) was found significantly more often than in controls (8%) [55].

Perhaps the most powerful evidence of a genetic linkage derives from the finding that in the only study of its type a high point prevalence of IGT was found in first-degree relatives (18.2%) and treatment-naïve schizophrenia subjects (10.5%) compared with healthy controls (0%) [60]. This study further emphasised the difficulty of carrying out studies in treatment-naïve subjects where cohort sizes are often modest and where selection of the most appropriate glucose parameter is difficult. Despite finding no significant differences between the cohorts in fasting glucose and HBA1c levels, both subjects and their relatives had elevated insulin levels and evidence of insulin resistance using HOMA-IR.

There are a number of studies that suggest a genetic overlap between diabetes and schizophrenia and bipolar disorder [61]. Some preliminary data from a small study in subjects with schizophrenia support a role of the MTHFR genotype in determining a predisposition to insulin resistance [62].

Glucose levels and other parameters have tended to show abnormalities in treatment-naïve subjects; however, not all studies are consistent in this finding [29, 63–66]. A consistent finding from the Dublin group has been elevation in glucose levels and increased abdominal fat in their treatment-naïve subjects [29, 42, 43]. The underlying mechanism has, however, remained undefined. Recently, it has been proposed that deficient IGF-1 levels may underlie insulin resistance in schizophrenia [67]. In a relatively large study of 88 subjects, subjects with schizophrenia had higher insulin levels and greater insulin resistance than controls with evidence of lower IGF-1 levels. Insulin levels were elevated even after controlling for cortisol. IGF-1 has been postulated as being involved in the pathogenesis of schizophrenia [68]. Similarly, in 45 first-episode subjects either treatment-naïve (n = 15) or receiving antipsychotic treatments for mostly less than 4 weeks with a normal baseline BMI of 24.29 (SD 4.06). Although the mean FPG was significantly greater than in the control cohort (p = 0.0467), there were no differences in insulin levels although they were numerically higher in the schizophrenia patients [64]. Categorical analyses showed elevated glucose (undefined but presumably IFG) in 2.5% of the patients and 0% of the controls. CAFÉ found no glucose differences amongst a series of atypical antipsychotics over a 1-year prospective study in first-episode subjects with schizophrenia.

Glucose Metabolism in Patients Treated with Antipsychotics

The putative role that antipsychotics may play with regard to changes in glucose metabolism has been discussed in a plethora of published data. Broadly, these fall into the categories of reviews and opinions [25, 26, 69, 70], pharmaco-epidemiological studies analysing existing data retrospectively [8, 71], and prospective trials in which glucose data have been collected. What is currently absent is a single RCT in which glucose metabolism is the primary endpoint of concern other than clamp studies.

In general terms, these have provided inconsistent findings for a number of clear reasons. Glucose abnormalities can only be detected by blood sampling and rates of screening for glucose have until recently been very low. Even in centres of excellence such as the Maudsley in London, UK, glucose screening was being undertaken in only 41% of inpatients receiving antipsychotics [11]. Furthermore, there are many confounders that should be adjusted for before attempting to compare rates of glucose changes in patients treated with antipsychotics including diagnosis, family history, weight, length of treatment, ethnicity, concomitant medications and gender, and many other potential confounders. Smoking has recently been defined as a major risk factor for type 2 diabetes [72] with a meta-analysis concluding that the risk of diabetes is increased by a relative risk (RR) of 1.61 (1.43–1.80) for heavy smokers (>20 cigarettes/day) with even former smokers having a RR of 1.23 (1.14–1.33). Rates of smoking in subjects with schizophrenia are high and cigarette consumption is also high [73–76]. Smoking is another confounder that has not been adjusted for in these studies.

Glucose Data from Prospective Clinical Trials

In 2004, the first review paper on glucose and schizophrenia data derived from prospective RCTs was published and concluded that at that time none of these data showed significant differences in changes in glucose parameters during treatment with different antipsychotics [77]. The paper further hypothesized that in some patients glucose elevations occur for reasons other than weight gain. Glucose data are collected during the majority of clinical trials and represent a routine safety parameter. The interest in glucose, insulin and glycosylated haemoglobin, however, mainly post-dates the currently marketed antipsychotics and hence did not represent a primary endpoint for any of their registration trials. Despite this, a great quantity of glucose data has been reported in many publications. In 2007, a systematic review of the then published glucose data reported that prospective glucose data were available from over 6,000 patients that participated in 22 RCTs [78]. The conclusion was that there were no consistent significant differences in changes in glucose parameters among patients treated with antipsychotics. Where any significant differences were reported, they were often in trials in which antipsychotics were used in doses 50–100% greater than the maximum licensed or labelled dose [79, 80] and trial methodologies and the reporting of the metabolic data made data interpretation complex. At present, there are now more than 30 RCTs with published glucose data and the data remain broadly similar in that no consistent significant differences between antipsychotics in individual RCTs have been reported. There are, however, a few studies that do show some differences, but these studies have unusual inclusion criteria. In an 8-week treatment-resistant study on schizophrenia where risperidone or placebo was added to clozapine treatment, the risperidone cohort had a greater increase in fasting glucose ($p = 0.04$) [81]. The baseline mean glucose in both cohorts was >5.6 mmol/l and thus in the range for IFG and the baseline mean PANSS was around 100. The significance of these data may also lie in the choice of parameter for analysis. Whereas there were no significant differences between the cohorts at 8 weeks in their mean glucose values the change from baseline was significant. During the study, a number of subjects (6/25 in the risperidone/clozapine cohort; 4/25 placebo/clozapine) had glucose levels >7 mmol/l at 8 weeks and were potentially diabetic.

Clinicians may have found this saga not only complex but difficult to follow. The complexities and weaknesses of the retrospective data need explanation [84] and the prospective data have not always been easily accessible. One of the earliest large comparative data sets was glucose data over 6 months derived from an RCT involving olanzapine and aripiprazole. These data were salient and important as they demonstrated that although significant weight gain was observed in the olanzapine cohort (3.6 kg) and a mean weight loss was observed in the aripiprazole cohort (0.9 kg), there was no significant difference in the incidence of new-onset diabetes between the two cohorts, i.e. 4.5 and 4.7%, respectively [77]. In these subjects, the non-fasting glucose had risen from <8.8 mmol/l at trial entry to >11.1 mmol/l. The data, however, were only published on a website before inclusion in the review paper [77]. Similarly, in the 2007 systematic review of prospective data [78] from the 22 studies, 16 were peer-reviewed papers, 4 posters from congresses, and 2 data from Internet sites. This paper also emphasised that FPG was reported in 16 studies and non-fasting in 7. The length of the reported studies is also important. Diabetes is recognised to be a slowly developing illness in which abnormalities in insulin resistance pre-date glucose changes by over 7 years. Only 3 studies were of at least 2 years follow-up which although long in terms of schizophrenia and psychiatry is short in glucose terms. A total of 15 studies were, however, longer than 5 months in duration. The conclusion from these prospective glucose data was that there did seem to be some consistency in that no study reported consistent glucose differences between patients treated with antipsychotics, which is in contrast to the plethora of different findings in retrospective studies [84]. Citrome et al. [85] have recently reviewed many of these retrospective studies and in addition to the inability to adjust for many confounders which makes their interpretation complex, their length of follow-up as measured by length of drug exposure at time of blood sampling is no longer than in the prospective studies. There is thus a difficult and complex task to analyze any potential role of treatment with antipsychotics in the change in glucose parameters if the traditional aetiology for diabetes is correct in schizophrenia and bipolar subjects. Some investigators may regard short-term glucose data as unhelpful to report.

In a recent study that reports glucose metabolism from an open-label 12- to 16-week study [86] from subjects receiving clozapine or amisulpride glucose data was not reported. The study found insulin resistance and plasma insulin levels to be elevated in the clozapine cohort.

What the trials have shown is that with regular glucose monitoring many new cases of diabetes and pre-diabetes will be found even in subjects currently receiving no antipsychotic medication. Aripiprazole and paliperidone are the most recent licensed antipsychotics in the UK and in their trial development placebo-controlled trials have been deemed essential by regulatory agencies. In the only study reporting on FPG levels in 2004 involving aripiprazole, over 6 months incident cases of abnormal glucose >6.1 mmol/l were measured in 5.5% subjects taking aripiprazole and 10.3% subjects on placebo [77]. Recent guidelines have thus correctly emphasised the need for regular glucose monitoring regardless of the specific antipsychotic treatment [30, 87]. Two fairly distinguished clinical trials, CAFÉ and CATIE studies [80, 82, 83], form part of the current evidence base. CAFÉ found no glucose differences between antipsychotics over a 1-year period.

The CATIE study has been the landmark study in the last 10 years because of its many facets, and is a long-term independent study sponsored by the NIMH [80]. Interpretation of the glucose data from the primary publication was complex as essentially the glucose levels were admixtures of fasting and random samples in the same patient at different time points and additionally glucose was not simply adjusted for length of treatments [88]. The CATIE group subsequently published their data on metabolic syndrome parameters and prevalence using fasting data only and have recently published further purely fasting glucose data [1]. Glucose parameters are best interpreted as categorical diagnoses (diabetes, IFT, IGT) and as mean changes from baseline, when comparing different antipsychotic treatment cohorts longitudinally. At entry to CATIE many subjects randomised to antipsychotic (37–48.4%) already met the NCEP criteria for metabolic syndrome [1, 48], and the glucose parameter of >5.6 mmol/l) was met by 25–35.1%. Utilising fasting glucose data only at baseline and 3 months there were no significant differences between the antipsychotic treatment groups. Rather surprisingly, the number of subjects receiving olanzapine who met the glucose criteria decreased from 35% to 27% (n = 74). Similarly, the mean fasting glucose changes at 3 and 9 months showed no significant glucose differences between the antipsychotics. A recent 4-week RCT evaluating ziprasidone and aripiprazole also reports small increases in the median FBG of 0.11 and 0.165 mmol/l, respectively [89].

Some studies suggest that patients treated with clozapine may have the highest potential risk of glucose elevation, though few data assess the severity of illness as a potential confounder. In a 10-year follow-up, 34% (n = 96) developed diabetes though the Kaplan-Meier estimate was 43% if all patients had taken clozapine for 10 years [90].

The difficulties of adequately interpreting these data remain complex without a clinical trial designed to follow-up the glucose and metabolic parameters in the long term. Although many studies report some degree of glucose elevation during treatment with most antipsychotics there are some that report decreases. In a small open-label randomised efficacy study of around 18 weeks' duration, significant glucose reductions were reported in all cohorts. The reason, however, is salient in that the authors report that baseline glucose levels were not fasting levels even though this was intended [91].

What Format of Glucose Testing Might Be Best in 2008?

The diagnosis of DM usually needs a FG appraisal and if this is feasible it should be undertaken. Recent groups reviewing this topic emphasise the pragmatic difficulty of obtaining fasting samples in SMI subjects and conclude that random samples may be feasible initially [25, 26, 28]. Certainly, the sensitivity and specificity between single FG and random glucose are not so major [27]. There are pragmatic difficulties with obtaining FPG in SMI subjects. In studies that require FPG, patients are often hospitalised [11, 29, 92]. There are clear concerns that it is difficult to accurately determine the fasting status of a patient. Despite these difficulties, investigators in Belgium report few difficulties in obtaining both FPG and undertaking OGTT. They report that without OGTT many cases of diabetes and IGT will be missed [18].

The OGTT, without doubt a good tool, is not practical in many cases despite good evidence that the sensitivity and specificity of DM diagnoses will be increased. Glycosylated haemoglobin continues to cause debate but recent data do suggest that it may be of value. The importance of re-testing in accordance with ADA and WHO definitions for the diagnosis of diabetes is clear.

A number of investigators have reported that subjects may not always remain in their original glucose diagnostic category [28]. In 8 subjects considered to be euglycaemic and found to have FPG >7 mmol/l and then re-tested, in only 50% (n = 4) was a diagnosis of diabetes ratified, 2 subjects falling into the 'pre-diabetes' group with IFG and the remaining 2 subjects having normal FPG levels.

The finding in one study that even when fasting samples are intended 75% will be non-fasting [28] further emphasises the importance of taking another look at random glucose. The IDF have recently brought out guidelines on the monitoring of glucose in diabetes and emphasise the importance of controlling post-meal hyperglycaemia [93]. A 2-hour post-meal sample <7.8 mmol/l is considered essential. The IDF consider post-meal hyperglycaemia to be a significant determinant for risk of cardiovascular disease (CVD) in subjects with normal glucose, IGT and diabetes [93]. Two large European and Asian studies (DECODE and DECODA) report 2-hour plasma glucose to be a better predictor of CVD and all-cause mortality than FPG [93]. The reality is also that without hospitalisation a 'fasting' sample may in some cases represent a random sample.

For the future, plasma 1,5-anhydroglucitol has been proposed as a marker for post-meal hyperglycaemia and has been available as an assay for a decade and reflects transient glucose elevations within only a few days.

Glucose Elevation and Wellness Programmes

There is clear evidence that in all forms of diabetes and pre-diabetes physical activity levels play an important role in treatment. There is also some evidence that levels of physical activity in subjects with all forms of severe mental illness are often very low and that these levels pre-date any antipsychotic treatment and weight gain [60, 75]. In the Spelman et al. [60] cohort, treatment-naïve subjects were doing significantly less physical activity than their first-degree relatives or controls. Furthermore, the discrepancy was greatest with moderate/vigorous exercise and had no relationship with BMI as the treatment-naïve cohort had significantly reduced BMIs ($p < 0.05$). Wellness programmes when applied with rigour can be very effective in reducing CVD risk factors in the SMI population. Over a 2-year period, the 'Well-Being Support Programme' reported a reduction in many CVD risk factors and a marked increase in levels of physical activity that were sustained throughout the 2 years [75, 76]. Although there seems little doubt that wellness and weight reduction programmes can be successful in some outpatients with SMI [94, 76, 74], some preliminary evidence that these programmes may also improve metabolic parameters [96, 97] in some patients is beginning to emerge. The choice of glucose parameter may be important in these relatively short-term studies. Mauri et al. [96] report a reduction in fasting insulin levels, insulin resistance (HOMA index) and improvement in insulin sensitivity but unchanged FPG in an olanzapine case series (49 subjects) predominantly with bipolar disorder treated for 24 weeks randomised to a psycho-educational programme for weight loss for either 12 or 24 weeks. Menza et al. [97] found a reduction in glycosylated haemoglobin over 1 year of from 5.35% to 5.11% ($n = 31$, $p = 0.001$) using a multi-modal weight control programme.

Conclusions

Prior to 2000, the published literature on any associations between mental illness and glucose was limited predominantly to case reports and small retrospective pharmacoepidemiological studies [84]. In the last 8 years, there has been a plethora of data driven mainly by clinicians' interest in schizophrenia and glucose [77, 78]. The complex relationship is only now starting to be partially clarified [63]. In 2003, data began to emerge describing glucose and metabolic disturbances present in treatment-naïve schizophrenia patients [29]. Since then the predominant questions asked have been related to the potential quantitative risks of glucose elevation associated with the illness of schizophrenia and during treatment with antipsychotic agents. These have proven complex and difficult questions to answer. Not only are long-term prospective metabolic data limited but the complexities of designing trials to minimise the frequently high dropout rates have proven restrictive. In 2008, there remains no single RCT designed with primary endpoints evaluating glucose endpoints.

Diabetes is highly prevalent in schizophrenia and bipolar disorders being diagnosed in 2–3 times as many subjects as the general population. Prevalence rates of 15% may be accurate. In addition, what is often wrongly termed 'pre-diabetes' is found in another 15%. Increased screening rates have led to increased prevalence and incidence rates being described in schizophrenia over the last decade but what is not known is if the incidence rate of DM in schizophrenia is rising faster than that in the general population but there is a possibility that it is. The epidemic of global obesity is associated with more DM in the general population and greater efforts are being made to increase glucose screening programmes. Around 20–30% of schizophrenia patients have a positive family history of DM and together with other genetic associations has led to certainty that schizophrenia and glucose are inextricably linked.

Patients treated with antipsychotics appear to have an increased risk of changes in glucose parameters. While relative risk estimates are inconsistent, the association between atypical antipsychotics and increases in glucose levels appears to fall on a continuum and olanzapine appears to have a greater association than some other atypical antipsychotics, the current UK opinion is that any differences between drugs are unlikely to be clinically relevant. The potential mechanisms whereby glucose elevations transpire are described but certainty is still lacking. Glucose data derived from animal models, human volunteers and schizophrenia patients has sometimes yielded conflicting science. The probability is that many mechanisms are involved. Where clarity is needed is in describing the cohort of patients who are most vulnerable to either or both of these mechanisms.

Over the next decade, we have a number of tasks. Firstly, we should ensure that regular glucose monitoring for all schizophrenia patients is the norm. Secondly, we should look to define the longer-term patterns of glucose elevation in patients treated with the numerous antipsychotics with greater precision. Data are starting to emerge showing that glucose abnormalities may be variable both in type and existence. Thirdly, we should aim to prevent the progression of glucose abnormalities through wellness and lifestyle intervention programmes. Finally, we should aim to significantly reduce the number of cases of DM and pre-diabetes.

The probability is that a final task may be unlikely to be achieved in the next decade and may require many decades of research. We should also aim to specifically quantify the CVD risk associated with elevations in glucose in comparison to the other CVD risk factors that are highly prevalent in schizophrenia. DM can be regarded as a risk factor for CVD in the general population; however, in a schizophrenia cohort already at a 3-fold increased risk of CVD to what greater extent does this elevate the risk?

References

1 Meyer JM, Davis VG, Goff DC, McEvoy JP, Nasrallah HA, Davis SM, Rosenheck RA, Daumit GL, Hsiao J, Swartz MS, Stroup TS, Lieberman JA: Change in metabolic syndrome parameters with antipsychotic treatment in the CATIE Schizophrenia Trial: Prospective data from phase 1. Schizophr Res 2008; 101:273–278.

2 Diabetes Atlas©, ed 3. International Diabetes Federation, 2006. (At /www.eatlas.idf.org/ accessed 1 March 2008.)

3 www.bhf.org

4 www.unitefordiabetes.org (accessed 1 March 2008).

5 Centers for Disease Control and Prevention. www.cdc.gov/nchs/about/major/nhis/released200303.htm

6 Kohen D: Diabetes mellitus and schizophrenia: historical perspective. Br J Psychiatry Suppl 2004;47:S64–S66.

7 Dixon L, Weiden P, Delahanty J: Prevalence and correlates of diabetes in national schizophrenia samples. Schizophr Bull 2000;2:903–912.

8 Sernyak MJ, Leslie DL, Alarcon RD, Losonczy MF, Rosenheck R: Association of diabetes mellitus with use of atypical neuroleptics in the treatment of schizophrenia. Am J Psychiatry 2002;159:561–566.

9 Bushe C, Holt R: Prevalence of diabetes and impaired glucose tolerance in patients with schizophrenia. Br J Psychiatry Suppl 2004;47:S67–S71.

10 Subramaniam M, Chong SA, Pek E: Diabetes mellitus and impaired glucose tolerance in patients with schizophrenia. Can J Psychiatry 2003;48:345–347.

11 Taylor D, Young C, Esop R, Paton C, Walwyn R: Testing for diabetes in hospitalised patients prescribed antipsychotic drugs. Br J Psychiatry 2004; 185:152–156.

12 Taylor D, Young C, Mohamed R, Paton C, Walwyn R: Undiagnosed impaired fasting glucose and diabetes mellitus amongst inpatients receiving antipsychotic drugs. J Psychopharmacol 2005;19: 182–186.

13 Citrome L, Jaffe A, Levine J, Allingham B, Robinson: Relationship between antipsychotic medication treatment and new cases of diabetes among psychiatric inpatients. Psychiatr Serv 2004;55:1006–1013.

14 Flegal KM, Carroll MD, Ogden CL, et al: Prevalence and trends in obesity among US adults, 1999–2000. JAMA 2002;288:1723–1727.

15 Smith RC, Lindenmayer JP, Bark N, Warner-Cohen J, Vaidhyanathaswamy S, Khandat A: Clozapine, risperidone, olanzapine, and conventional antipsychotic drug effects on glucose, lipids, and leptin in schizophrenic patients. Int J Neuropsychopharmacol 2005;8:183–194.

16 Citrome L, Jaffe A, Levine J, et al: Incidence, prevalence, and surveillance for diabetes in New York State psychiatric hospitals, 1997–2004. Psychiatr Serv 2006; 57:1132–1139.

17 National Center for Chronic Disease Prevention and Health Promotion. Incidence of diabetes. 2005 //www.cdc.gov/diabetes

18 van Winkel R, De Hert M, Wampers M, Van Eyck D, Hanssens L, Scheen A, Peuskens J: Major changes in glucose metabolism, including new-onset diabetes, within 3 months after initiation of or switch to atypical antipsychotic medication in patients with schizophrenia and schizoaffective disorder. J Clin Psychiatry 2008;69:472–479.

19 van Winkel R, De Hert M, Van Eyck D, Hanssens L, Wampers M, Scheen A, Peuskens J: Screening for diabetes and other metabolic abnormalities in patients with schizophrenia and schizoaffective disorder: evaluation of incidence and screening methods. J Clin Psychiatry 2006;67:1493–1500.

20 Lambert BL, Cunningham FE, Miller DR, Dalack GW, Hur K: Diabetes risk associated with use of olanzapine, quetiapine, and risperidone in veterans health administration patients with schizophrenia. Am J Epidemiol 2006;164:672–681.

21 Leslie DL, Rosenheck RA: Incidence of newly diagnosed diabetes attributable to atypical antipsychotic medications. Am J Psychiatry 2004;161:1709–1711.

22 Miller EA, Leslie DL, Rosenheck RA: Incidence of new-onset diabetes mellitus among patients receiving atypical neuroleptics in the treatment of mental illness: evidence from a privately insured population. J Nerv Ment Dis 2005;193:387–395.

23 Lambert MT, Copeland LA, Sampson N, Duffy SA: New-onset type-2 diabetes associated with atypical antipsychotic medications. Prog Neuropsychopharmacol Biol Psychiatry 2006;30:919–923.

24 De Hert M, van Winkel R, Van Eyck D, Hanssens L, Wampers M, Scheen A, Peuskens J: Prevalence of diabetes, metabolic syndrome and metabolic abnormalities in schizophrenia over the course of the illness: a cross-sectional study. Clin Pract Epidemiol Ment Health 2006;2:14.

25 Expert Group: 'Schizophrenia and Diabetes 2003' Expert Consensus Meeting, Dublin, 3–4 October 2003:consensus summary. Br J Psychiatry 2004;184 (suppl 47):S112–S114.

26 Expert Group: Metabolic and lifestyle issues and severe mental illness – new connections to well-being? Expert consensus meeting Dublin 2005. J Psychopharm 2005;19(6 suppl):118–122.

27 Gough S, Peveler R: Diabetes and its prevention: pragmatic solutions for people with schizophrenia. Br J Psychiatry Suppl 2004;47:S106–S111.

28 Sernyak MJ, Gulanski B, Rosenheck R: Undiagnosed hyperglycemia in patients treated with atypical antipsychotics. J Clin Psychiatry 2005; 66:1463–1467.

29 Ryan MC, Collins P, Thakore JH: Impaired fasting glucose tolerance in first-episode, drug-naive patients with schizophrenia. Am J Psychiatry 2003; 160:284–289.

30 The management of bipolar disorder in adults, children and adolescents, in primary and secondary care. NICE Bipolar Guidelines, 2006. www.nice.org.uk (accessed 9 March 2008).

31 Cassidy F, Ahearn E, Carroll BJ: Elevated frequency of diabetes mellitus in hospitalized manic-depressive patients. Am J Psychiatry 1999;156:1417–1420.

32 Regenold WT, Thapar RK, Marano C, et al: Increased prevalence of type 2 diabetes mellitus among psychiatric inpatients with bipolar I affective and schizoaffective disorders independent of psychotropic drug use. J Affect Disord 2002;70:19–26.

33 Yumru M, Savas HA, Kurt E, Kaya MC, Selek S, Savas E, Oral ET, Atagun I: Atypical antipsychotics related metabolic syndrome in bipolar patients. J Affect Disord 2007;98:247–252.

34 Fagiolini A, Frank E, Scott JA, Turkin S, Kupfer DJ: Metabolic syndrome in bipolar disorder: findings from the Bipolar Disorder Center for Pennsylvanians. Bipolar Disord 2005;7:424–430.

35 Goethe JW, Szarek BL, Caley CF, Woolley SB: Signs and symptoms associated with the metabolic syndrome in psychiatric inpatients receiving antipsychotics: a retrospective chart review. J Clin Psychiatry 2007;68:22–28.
36 Willis T: Diabetes: A Medical Odyssey. New York, Tuckahoe, 1971.
37 Lustman PJ, Clouse RE: Depression in diabetic patients: the relationship between mood and glycemic control. J Diabetes Compl 2005;19:113–122.
38 Anderson RJ, Freedland KE, Clouse RE, Lustman PJ: The prevalence of comorbid depression in adults with diabetes: a meta-analysis. Diabetes Care 2001; 24:1069–1078.
39 Lustman PJ, Clouse RE, Freedland KE: Management of major depression in adults with diabetes: implications of recent clinical trials. Semin Clin Neuropsychiatry 1998;3:102–114.
40 Lustman PJ, Anderson RJ, Freedland KE, de Groot M, Carney RM, Clouse RE: Depression and poor glycemic control: a meta-analytic review of the literature. Diabetes Care 2000;23:934–942.
41 Haro JM, Suarez D, Novick D, Brown J, Usall J, Naber D, SOHO Study Group: Three-year antipsychotic effectiveness in the outpatient care of schizophrenia: observational versus randomized studies results. Eur Neuropsychopharmacol 2007;17:235–244.
42 Thakore JH, Mann JN, Vlahos I, Martin A, Reznek R: Increased visceral fat distribution in drug-naive and drug-free patients with schizophrenia. Int J Obes Relat Metab Disord 2002;26:137–141.
43 Ryan MC, Flanagan S, Kinsella U, Keeling F, Thakore JH: The effects of atypical antipsychotics on visceral fat distribution in first episode, drug-naive patients with schizophrenia. Life Sci 20045;74:1999–2008. Erratum in: Life Sci 2004;75:2851.
44 Ader M, Garvey WT, Phillips LS, Nemeroff CB, Gharabawi G, Mahmoud R, Greenspan A, Berry SA, Musselman DL, Morein J, Zhu Y, Mao L, Bergman RN: Ethnic heterogeneity in glucoregulatory function during treatment with atypical antipsychotics in patients with schizophrenia. J Psychiatr Res 2008;42:1076–1085.
45 Sacher J, Mossaheb N, Spindelegger C, Klein N, Geiss-Granadia T, Sauermann R, Lackner E, Joukhadar C, Müller M, Kasper S: Effects of olanzapine and ziprasidone on glucose tolerance in healthy volunteers. Neuropsychopharmacology 2008;33: 1633–1641.
46 Henderson DC, Cagliero E, Copeland PM, Borba CP, Evins E, Hayden D, Weber MT, Anderson EJ, Allison DB, Daley TB, Schoenfeld D, Goff DC: Glucose metabolism in patients with schizophrenia treated with atypical antipsychotic agents: a frequently sampled intravenous glucose tolerance test and minimal model analysis. Arch Gen Psychiatry 2005;62:19–28.
47 Henderson DC, Copeland PM, Borba CP, Daley TB, Nguyen DD, Cagliero E, Evins AE, Zhang H, Hayden DL, Freudenreich O, Cather C, Schoenfeld DA, Goff DC: Glucose metabolism in patients with schizophrenia treated with olanzapine or quetiapine: a frequently sampled intravenous glucose tolerance test and minimal model analysis. J Clin Psychiatry 2006;67:789–797.
48 McEvoy J, Meyer M, Goff D, Nasrallah H, Davis S, Sullivan L, Meltzer HY, Hsiao J, Stroup TS, Lieberman JA: Prevalence of the metabolic syndrome in patients with schizophrenia: baseline results from the Clinical Antipsychotic Trials of Intervention Effectiveness (CATIE) schizophrenia trial and comparison with national estimates from NHANES III. Schizophr Res 2005;80:19–32.
49 Sowell MO, Mukhopadhyay N, Cavazzoni P, Shankar S, Steinberg HO, Breier A, Beasley CM Jr, Dananberg J: Hyperglycemic clamp assessment of insulin secretory responses in normal subjects treated with olanzapine, risperidone, or placebo. J Clin Endocrinol Metab 2002;87:2918–2923.
50 Haupt DW, Fahnestock PA, Flavin KA, Schweiger JA, Stevens A, Hessler MJ, Maeda J, Yingling M, Newcomer JW: Adiposity and insulin sensitivity derived from intravenous glucose tolerance tests in antipsychotic-treated patients. Neuropsychopharmacology 2007;32:2561–2569.
51 Chiu CC, Chen KP, Liu HC, Lu ML: The early effect of olanzapine and risperidone on insulin secretion in atypical-naïve schizophrenic patients. J Clin Psychopharmacol 2006;26:504–507.
52 Ader M, Kim SP, Catalano KJ, Ionut V, Hucking K, Richey JM, Kabir M, Bergman RN: Metabolic dysregulation with atypical antipsychotics occurs in the absence of underlying disease: a placebo-controlled study of olanzapine and risperidone in dogs. Diabetes 2005;54:862–871.
53 Hardy TA, Meyers AL, Yu J, Shankar SS, Steinberg HO, Porksen NK: Acute insulin response and beta-cell compensation in normal subjects treated with olanzapine or risperidone for 2 weeks. Diabetes Care 2007;30:157–158.
54 Wu MK, Huang CY, Liou YJ, Wang CK, Lee SD: Glucose-insulin homeostasis, lipid profiles and GH-IGF-IGFBP axis in clozapine-treated schizophrenic obesity versus non-psychiatric obesity. Int J Obes (Lond) 2008;32:436–442.
55 Fernandez-Egea E, Miller B, Bernardo M, Donner T, Kirkpatrick B: Parental history of type 2 diabetes in patients with nonaffective psychosis. Schizophr Res 2008;98:302–306.
56 Mukherjee S, Schnur DB, Reddy R: Family history of type 2 diabetes in schizophrenic patients. Lancet 1989;i:495.

57 Mackin P, Bishop D, Watkinson H, Gallagher P, Ferrier IN: Metabolic disease and cardiovascular risk in people treated with antipsychotics in the community. Br J Psychiatry 2007;191:23–29.
58 Valdez R, Yoon PW, Liu T, Khoury MJ: Family history and prevalence of diabetes in the U.S. population: the 6-year results from the National Health and Nutrition Examination Survey (1999–2004). Diabetes Care 2007;30:2517–2522.
59 Mata-Cases M, Fernández-Bertolín E, Cos-Claramunt X, García-Durán M, Mateu-Gelabert T, Pareja-Rossell C, Pujol-Ribera E: Incidence of type 2 diabetes and its diagnosis process in the decade 1991–2000 in a primary health care centre. Gac Sanit 2006;20:124–131.
60 Spelman LM, Walsh PI, Sharifi N, Collins P, Thakore JH: Impaired glucose tolerance in first-episode drug-naïve patients with schizophrenia. Diabet Med 2007;24: 481–485.
61 Gough SC, O'donovan MC: Clustering of metabolic comorbidity in schizophrenia: a genetic contribution? J Psychopharmacol 2005;19(suppl):47–55.
62 Ellingrod VL, Miller del D, Taylor SF, Moline J, Holman T, Kerr J: Metabolic syndrome and insulin resistance in schizophrenia patients receiving antipsychotics genotyped for the methylenetetrahydrofolate reductase (MTHFR) 677C/T and 1298A/C variants. Schizophr Res 2008;98:47–54.
63 Holt RI, Bushe C, Citrome L: Diabetes and schizophrenia 2005:are we any closer to understanding the link? J Psychopharmacol 2005;19(suppl):56–65.
64 Graham KA, Cho H, Brownley KA, Harp JB: Early treatment-related changes in diabetes and cardiovascular disease risk markers in first episode psychosis subjects. Schizophr Res 2008;101:287–294.
65 Arranz B, Rosel P, Ramírez N, Dueñas R, Fernández P, Sanchez JM, Navarro MA, San L: Insulin resistance and increased leptin concentrations in noncompliant schizophrenia patients but not in antipsychotic-naive first-episode schizophrenia patients. J Clin Psychiatry 2004;65:1335–1342.
66 Zhang ZJ, Yao ZJ, Liu W, Fang Q, Reynolds GP: Effects of antipsychotics on fat deposition and changes in leptin and insulin levels: magnetic resonance imaging study of previously untreated people with schizophrenia. Br J Psychiatry 2004;184: 58–62.
67 Venkatasubramanian G, Chittiprol S, Neelakantachar N, Naveen MN, Thirthall J, Gangadhar BN, Shetty KT: Insulin and insulin-like growth factor-1 abnormalities in antipsychotic-naive schizophrenia. Am J Psychiatry 2007;164:1557–1560.
68 Gunnell D, Holly JM: Hypothesis: do insulin-like growth factors underlie associations of birth complications, fetal and pre-adult growth with schizophrenia? Schizophr Res 2004;71:191–193.
69 American Diabetes Association; American Psychiatric Association; American Association of Clinical Endocrinologists; North American Association for the Study of Obesity: Consensus development conference on antipsychotic drugs and obesity and diabetes. Diabetes Care 2004;27: 596–601.
70 Barnett AH, Mackin P, Chaudhry I, Farooqi A, Gadsby R, Heald A, Hill J, Millar H, Peveler R, Rees A, Singh V, Taylor D, Vora J, Jones P: Minimising metabolic and cardiovascular risk in schizophrenia: diabetes, obesity and dyslipidaemia. J Psychopharmacol 2007;21:357–373.
71 Koro CE, Fedder DO, L'Italien GJ, et al: Assessment of independent effect of olanzapine and risperidone on risk of diabetes among patients with schizophrenia: population based nested case control study. Br Med J 2002;325:243–248.
72 Willi C, Bodenmann P, Ghali WA, Faris PD, Cornuz J: Active smoking and the risk of type 2 diabetes: a systematic review and meta-analysis. JAMA 2007;298:2654–2664.
73 McCreadie RG, Scottish Schizophrenia Lifestyle Group: Diet, smoking and cardiovascular risk in people with schizophrenia: descriptive study. Br J Psychiatry 2003;183:534–539.
74 Bushe C, Haddad P, Peveler R, Pendlebury J: The role of lifestyle interventions and weight management in schizophrenia. J Psychopharmacol 2005; 19(suppl):28–35.
75 Smith S, Yeomans D, Bushe CJ, Eriksson C, Harrison T, Holmes R, Mynors-Wallis L, Oatway H, Sullivan G: A well-being programme in severe mental illness: baseline findings in a UK cohort. Int J Clin Pract 2007;61:1971–1978.
76 Smith S, Yeomans D, Bushe CJ, Eriksson C, Harrison T, Holmes R, Mynors-Wallis L, Oatway H, Sullivan G: A well-being programme in severe mental illness. Reducing risk for physical ill-health: a post-programme service evaluation at 2 years. Eur Psychiatry 2007;22:413–418.
77 Bushe CJ, Leonard BE: Blood glucose and schizophrenia: a systematic review of prospective randomized clinical trials. J Clin Psychiatry 2007;68: 1682–1690.
78 Bushe C, Leonard B: Association between atypical antipsychotic agents and type 2 diabetes: review of prospective clinical data. Br J Psychiatry Suppl 2004; 47:S87–S93.
79 Lindenmayer JP, Czobor P, Volavka J, Citrome L, Sheitman B, McEvoy JP, Cooper TB, Chakos M, Lieberman JA: Changes in glucose and cholesterol levels in patients with schizophrenia treated with typical or atypical antipsychotics. Am J Psychiatry 2003;160:290–296.

80 Lieberman JA, Stroup TS, McEvoy JP, Swartz MS, Rosenheck RA, Perkins DO, Keefe RSE, Davis SM, Davis CE, Lebowitz BD, Severe J, Hsiao JK: Effectiveness of antipsychotic drugs in patients with chronic schizophrenia. N Engl J Med 2005;353:1209–1223.

81 Honer WG, Thornton AE, Chen EY, Chan RC, Wong JO, Bergmann A, Falkai P, Pomarol-Clotet E, McKenna PJ, Stip E, Williams R, MacEwan GW, Wasan K, Procyshyn R, Clozapine and Risperidone Enhancement (CARE) Study Group: Clozapine alone versus clozapine and risperidone with refractory schizophrenia. N Engl J Med 2006;354:472–482.

82 Olanzapine USA Label 2008.

83 McEvoy JP, Lieberman JA, Perkins DO, Hamer RM, Gu H, Lazarus A, Sweitzer D, Olexy C, Weiden P, Strakowski SD: Efficacy and tolerability of olanzapine, quetiapine and risperidone in the treatment of early psychosis: a randomised, double blind 52 week comparison. Am J Psychiatry 2007;164:1050–1060.

84 Haddad PM: Antipsychotics and diabetes: review of non-prospective data. Br J Psychiatry Suppl 2004;47:S80–S86.

85 Citrome LL, Holt RI, Zachry WM, Clewell JD, Orth PA, Karagianis JL, Hoffmann VP: Risk of treatment-emergent diabetes mellitus in patients receiving antipsychotics. Ann Pharmacother 2007;41:1593–1603.

86 Rettenbacher MA, Hummer M, Hofer A, Baumgartner S, Ebenbichler C, Edlinger M, Kemmler G, Lechleitner M, Wolfgang Fleischhacker W: Alterations of glucose metabolism during treatment with clozapine or amisulpride: results from a prospective 16-week study. J Psychopharmacol 2007;21:400–404.

87 Taylor D, Paton C, Kerwin R: The South London and Maudsley NHS Foundation Trust and Oxleas NHS Foundation Trust Prescribing Guidelines, ed 9. Informa Healthcare 2007.

88 Haddad P, Dursun SM: Selecting antipsychotics in schizophrenia: lessons from CATIE. J Psychopharmacol 2006;20:332–334.

89 Zimbroff D, Warrington L, Loebel A, Yang R, Siu C: Comparison of ziprasidone and aripiprazole in acutely ill patients with schizophrenia or schizoaffective disorder: a randomized, double-blind, 4-week study. Int Clin Psychopharmacol 2007;22: 363–370.

90 Henderson DC, Nguyen DD, Copeland PM, Hayden DL, Borba CP, Louie PM, Freudenreich O, Evins AE, Cather C, Goff DC: Clozapine, diabetes mellitus, hyperlipidemia, and cardiovascular risks and mortality: results of a 10-year naturalistic study. J Clin Psychiatry 2005;66:1116–1121.

91 Suzuki T, Uchida H, Watanabe K, Nomura K, Takeuchi H, Tomita M, Tsunoda K, Nio S, Den R, Manki H, Tanabe A, Yagi G, Kashima H: How effective is it to sequentially switch among olanzapine, quetiapine and risperidone? A randomized, open-label study of algorithm-based antipsychotic treatment to patients with symptomatic schizophrenia in the real-world clinical setting. Psychopharmacology (Berl) 2007;195:285–295.

92 Paton C, Esop R, Young C, Taylor D: Obesity, dyslipidaemias and smoking in an inpatient population treated with antipsychotic drugs. Acta Psychiatr Scand 2004;110:299–305.

93 www.idf.org: Guideline for management of post-meal glucose 2007 (accessed 25 Feb 2008).

94 Pendlebury J, Bushe CJ, Wildgust HJ, Holt RI: Long-term maintenance of weight loss in patients with severe mental illness through a behavioural treatment programme in the UK. Acta Psychiatr Scand 2007;115:286–294.

95 Lee SJ, Choi EJ, Kwon JS: A naturalistic multicenter trial of a 12-week weight management program for overweight and obese patients with schizophrenia or schizoaffective disorder. J Clin Psychiatry 2008;69:555–562.

96 Mauri M, Simoncini M, Castrogiovanni S, Iovieno N, Cecconi D, Dell'Agnello G, Quadrigli M, Rossi A, Donda P, Fagiolini A, Cassano GB: A psychoeducational program for weight loss in patients who have experienced weight gain during antipsychotic treatment with olanzapine. Pharmacopsychiatry 2008;41:17–23.

97 Menza M, Vreeland B, Minsky S, Gara M, Radler DR, Sakowitz M: Managing atypical antipsychotic-associated weight gain: 12-month data on a multimodal weight control program. J Clin Psychiatry 2004;65:471–477.

Chris Bushe, MB, BS
Lilly UK, Lilly House, Priestley Road
Basingstoke, Hampshire, RG24 9NL (UK)
Tel. +44 1256 775 971, Fax +44 1256 775 858, E-Mail bushe_chris@lilly.com

Thakore J, Leonard BE (eds): Metabolic Effects of Psychotropic Drugs.
Mod Trends Pharmacopsychiatry. Basel, Karger, 2009, vol 26, pp 66–81

Screening for Diabetes and Cardiovascular Risk Factors in People with Serious Mental Illness

Richard I.G. Holt[a] · Robert C. Peveler[b]

[a]Endocrinology and Metabolism Sub-division, Developmental Origins of Health and Disease Division, and [b]Clinical Neurosciences Division, School of Medicine, University of Southampton, Southampton, UK

Abstract

Physical health care has been a frequently neglected yet essential component of the holistic care of people with schizophrenia or bipolar illness. The rates of diabetes and cardiovascular disease are increased 2- to 3 fold compared with the general population. This, coupled with lower rates of diagnosis, has led to calls for screening for diabetes and cardiovascular disease in individuals with serious mental illness. The UK national screening committee has produced criteria for appraising the viability, effectiveness and appropriateness of a screening programme. Most of these criteria are met for screening for diabetes and cardiovascular disease risk factors. As there are no formal screening programmes, some criteria are not satisfied. There is a clear imperative to introduce screening for diabetes and CVD risk factors but at the same time, further research is needed to evaluate these interventions.

Physical health care has been a frequently neglected yet essential component of the holistic care of the person with serious mental illness (SMI). The standardised mortality ratio is increased three fold in those with schizophrenia and life expectancy is reduced by 10–20 years [1]. While suicide and traumatic death are important contributors to premature mortality and have the highest relative risk compared with the general population, mortality rates associated with physical illness are doubled and account for around three quarters of all deaths in people with schizophrenia. Cardiovascular disease is the commonest cause of death accounting for 30–50% of all deaths [2]. Mortality rates are also increased in those with affective disorders, with depression being as strong a risk factor for cardiovascular disease as smoking.

The causes of excess physical illness are multifactorial and are likely to include both genetic and environmental factors, as well as disease-specific and treatment effects.

Table 1. Degree to which screening for diabetes and cardiovascular disease meets the UK National Screening Committee criteria

Criterion	Diabetes	CVD
Important health problem	✓	✓
Natural history understood	✓	✓
Primary prevention implemented	x/✓	✓
Simple, safe, precise and validated screening test	✓	✓
Distribution and cut-off test values agreed	✓	✓
Acceptability of test	?	?
Need for further diagnostic investigation agreed	✓	✓
Effective treatment	✓	✓
Who should receive treatment	✓	✓
Optimal clinical management and patient outcomes	x/✓	x/✓
Screening shown to be effective	x	x
Acceptability of screening programme	?	?
Potential for harm	?	?
Cost effectiveness	x/✓	x/✓
Quality assurance	x	x
Adequate staffing	✓	✓
Other options considered	✓	✓
Information about screening	x/✓	x/✓
Widening of screening programme	✓	✓

The physical health care provided may also be of poorer quality as people with SMI may find it harder to describe and discuss physical symptoms, and such symptoms may be ignored by health care professionals, or else mistaken for manifestations of the mental illness. Lack of access to physical health services creates a further barrier to those with mental illness.

The case for screening may be stronger in people with SMI where the rates of physical illness are higher and are coupled with lower diagnosis. This has led several bodies to recommend screening for both diabetes and cardiovascular risk factors in people with SMI [3–10]. The aim of this review is to determine to what extent these recommendations are justified by considering them with reference to the UK national screening committee criteria for appraising the viability, effectiveness and appropriateness of a screening programme (table 1) [11]. Ideally, all criteria should be met before screening for a condition is initiated. At present, most screening is opportunistic and formal screening programmes do not exist.

Pubmed and other electronic databases were searched to identify articles that addressed this issue by including the key words: diabetes, cardiovascular disease, psychosis, schizophrenia, bipolar illness and screening.

The Condition

The condition should be an important health problem

Diabetes

Diabetes was thought to affect 189 million people worldwide in 2003. The prevalence is increasing on all continents and it is estimated that by 2025, at least 324 million will have diabetes. Diabetes is associated with considerable premature mortality and morbidity primarily through its long term complications which include cardiovascular disease and the microvascular complications of nephropathy, neuropathy and retinopathy [12]. 16% of all new patients needing renal replacement therapy have diabetes. 15% of people with diabetes develop foot ulcers as a result of diabetic neuropathy and peripheral vascular disease, and of these 5–15% need amputations. Diabetes is the commonest cause of non-traumatic lower limb amputation. Diabetic retinopathy is the commonest cause of blindness in people of working age. Diabetes is associated with a 2- to 3-fold increase in cardiovascular disease. In addition to its personal cost, diabetes accounts for 5–10% of the total health care spend in the UK [13].

Among people with SMI, rates of diabetes are increased 2- to 3-fold and 10–15% of people with SMI living in the Western world are affected [14].

Cardiovascular Disease

Cardiovascular disease (CVD) includes coronary heart disease, cerebrovascular disease and peripheral vascular disease [15]. It is the commonest cause of death in developed countries and its prevalence is also rapidly increasing in developing countries. In the UK, there were over 124,000 deaths from coronary heart disease, almost 61,000 deaths from stroke and 18,000 deaths from other circulatory diseases in 2000. The next commonest cause of death was respiratory disease, accounting for 103,000 deaths. In addition to the mortality associated with cardiovascular disease, there is considerable morbidity, resulting from stroke, angina and heart failure.

The cost of CVD to the UK economy in 2004 was GBP 29.1 billion, with coronary heart disease and cerebrovascular disease accounting for 29 and 27% of the total, respectively. Health care costs accounted for 60% of the cost and productivity losses due to mortality and morbidity accounted for 23% [15]. While 54% of the health costs were for hospital care and 32% for drug costs, less than 1% of that amount was spent on CVD prevention. This huge health cost has led to several government initiatives to reduce this burden on the National Health Service such as the National Service Framework (NSF) for Cardiovascular Disease [15] and the General Medical Services contract for primary care that specifically pays general practitioners to identify and treat cardiovascular risk factors [16].

The prevalence of CVD is increased in people with SMI. In a recent retrospective cohort study of 46,136 people with SMI, the rates of CVD in those under 50 years old were 3.6-fold higher in those with schizophrenia and 2.1-fold higher in people with bipolar disorder [2]. The risk of stroke was 2.9- and 3.3-fold higher in people with schizophrenia and bipolar illness respectively. Both sexes were equally affected and traditional risk factors such as smoking and social deprivation did not fully explain this increase. Although the use of antipsychotic medication was associated with coronary heart disease, the risk was greater in those who never used antipsychotics.

The epidemiology and natural history of the condition, including development from latent to declared disease, should be adequately understood and there should be a detectable risk factor, disease marker, latent period or early symptomatic stage

Diabetes

Type 2 diabetes accounts for over 90% of all cases of diabetes [12]. The pathogenesis of type 2 diabetes involves two main pathological abnormalities, insulin resistance and pancreatic β-cell failure. One model of the natural history proposes that as insulin resistance worsens, initially there is a compensatory increase in insulin secretion to meet the physiological requirements, but a point is reached where the demands exceed β-cell secretory capacity and thereafter insulin secretion falls. This gradual decline in insulin secretion leads to an insidious rise in both fasting and post-prandial glucose, which may remain asymptomatic for as long as a decade during the early stages of the disease. During this time, however, the hyperglycaemia is not innocuous, as 50% of people with type 2 diabetes already have microvascular complications at the time of diagnosis. Similarly asymptomatic diabetes may contribute to macrovascular disease as diabetes is commonly diagnosed on the coronary care unit [12].

The risk factors for type 2 diabetes have been well defined and are divided into two main groups depending on whether they are modifiable or not (table 2). The high rates of diabetes among people with SMI have meant that several bodies have identified this as an independent risk factor for diabetes [7, 9].

Given the long asymptomatic period in the early natural history of diabetes, within the general population it is estimated that for every two people with known diabetes, there is another person with undiagnosed diabetes [7]. Among people with SMI, the proportion of people with undiagnosed diabetes is much higher and may be as high as 70% of all cases [14].

Table 2. Risk factors for diabetes and cardiovascular disease

	Diabetes	Cardiovascular disease
Un-modifiable	Family history Low birth weight Non-white European ethnic background Ageing	Family history of premature cardiovascular disease Male gender Ageing Non-white European ethnic background Low birth weight Previous CV event
Modifiable	Obesity Diet Physical inactivity SMI	Dyslipidaemia (increased total and LDL cholesterol and decreased HDL cholesterol) Hypertension Obesity Diabetes Physical inactivity Smoking Metabolic syndrome

Cardiovascular Disease

There is a clear understanding of the natural history of the development of CVD. The first changes are seen during the teens when fatty streaks appear in the aorta. Increased intimal medial thickness, which can be detected in the carotid arteries, is an early sign of cardiovascular disease. Atherosclerotic plaques develop with time and rupture of these is usually associated with a clinical presentation that is dependent on the site of the lesion. When this occurs within a coronary artery, it precipitates a myocardial infarction, while rupture in a cerebral vessel leads to a stroke. Although narrowing of the arteries *per se* may also cause clinical symptoms such as angina (coronary arteries) or intermittent claudication (peripheral arteries), atherosclerosis is frequently asymptomatic during the early phases of the natural history and the first presentation may be dramatic or even fatal.

The risk factors for cardiovascular disease are well recognised and like those for diabetes can be divided into unmodifiable and modifiable risk factors (table 2). The metabolic syndrome, which is defined by a cluster of cardiovascular risk factors, is associated with around a 75% increased risk of cardiovascular disease. How the presence of this should be used to aid the identification of those at highest risk remains the subject of debate.

As the first presentation may occur without warning and may have serious consequences, several groups have attempted to create risk engines to assess an individual's risk for a cardiovascular event over a 10-year period, the most frequently used of which is based on the Framingham study [17].

All the cost-effective primary prevention interventions should have been implemented as far as practicable

Diabetes

There is good trial evidence that diabetes can be prevented or at least delayed by lifestyle intervention. Studies from China, Finland and the USA have all shown that dietary modification and increased physical activity can reduce the incidence of diabetes in individuals at high risk of diabetes [18] but the challenge for health care professionals has been to implement these findings into clinical practice. There is considerable nihilism about the possibility of lifestyle modification in people with SMI but recent studies have suggested that this is possible [19]. Although these studies have concentrated on diet or weight as an outcome rather than diabetes, the close relation between obesity and diabetes suggests that prevention of diabetes should be possible in this patient group.

In addition to lifestyle intervention, several pharmacological measures have been shown to be effective in preventing diabetes including metformin, acarbose (an α-glucosidase inhibitor), orlistat and the PPARγ agonists, troglitazone and rosiglitazone [18]. Their place in the routine prevention of diabetes has not been fully determined but in general their effect size is smaller than lifestyle modification and any benefit needs to be balanced against the costs and potential side effects. Nevertheless, pharmacological treatment may have a place for those at particularly high risk where lifestyle modification is either unfeasible or has been tried and failed.

While lifestyle modification interventions have been implemented by some mental health care providers, this is by no means universal and further development is needed to ensure that all people with SMI have access to lifestyle programmes. Although lifestyle and pharmacological interventions are effective in reducing diabetes, they do not prevent all cases of diabetes because they cannot affect unmodifiable risk factors and so even in the absence of universal lifestyle modification, screening may still be justified.

Cardiovascular Disease

The most important non-pharmacological intervention to reduce CVD is facilitation of smoking cessation, and there is some evidence to support the effectiveness of this [20]. Many health care providers now offer support to help individuals quit smoking and these programmes may also include the use of nicotine replacement. Although epidemiological studies would suggest that measures to increase physical activity, change diet and lose weight are also important, it is believed that pharmacological therapy is the most important measure to reduce CVD events in high risk subjects and the purpose of the screening test is to identify those who would benefit most from these interventions [15].

Table 3. Specificity and sensitivity for various screening methods for type 2 diabetes

Test	Specificity, %	Sensitivity, %
Fasting blood glucose	84–99	40–95
Random blood glucose	92–98	50–69
HbA_{1c}	79–100	35–98

There are well-powered and conducted studies that have shown convincingly that the use of lipid lowering agents (predominantly statins), aspirin, blood pressure agents will reduce cardiovascular events [15].

The Test

There should be a simple, safe, precise and validated screening test

Diabetes

There is considerable debate about the optimal screening test for diabetes but all of the available tests are simple and safe [21]. The gold standard investigation is the 75-gram oral glucose tolerance test, but this is impractical as a screening tool for the general population and for people with SMI in particular. The requirement for an overnight fast followed by two samples over a 2-hour period may create cost and logistical difficulties, and when population wide screening for diabetes was considered, it was realized that this test would be too onerous for most general practices. By contrast, Belgian psychiatrists have employed this test with success, perhaps reflecting differences in the systems of provision of care [22].

Alternatives to the glucose tolerance test include fasting glucose, random glucose and glycosylated haemoglobin estimations (table 3). The fasting glucose is recommended by Diabetes UK and American Diabetes Association as the test of choice but it will miss a number of cases where post-prandial hyperglycaemia is the only abnormality [7]. One of the earliest pathophysiological abnormalities in type 2 diabetes is the loss of early phase insulin secretion and this may lead to isolated post-prandial hyperglycaemia. Furthermore, diabetes in women and non-Caucasian people is more likely to be missed with a fasting glucose. Another disadvantage of a fasting sample is the extra behavioural demand on the person undergoing the test, which may be harder to meet for people with SMI.

The sensitivity and specificity of a random glucose sample is similar to a fasting glucose but the small loss of sensitivity is outweighed by the convenience of the test which can be undertaken at any time [21]. In an outpatient group, where the timing of last meal may not be reliably assessed, this test offers a pragmatic compromise between diagnostic accuracy and practicality.

Glyosylated haemoglobin (HbA_{1c}) has low sensitivity when used alone (approximately 35%) and therefore is not recommended to be used in isolation because of the large number of missed cases. When used together with a blood glucose concentration, the sensitivity improves up to 98%. Coupled with a specificity rate of 79–100%, the addition of HbA_{1c} provides useful information where it is not clear whether an individual has fasted or not [21].

Previously glycosuria has been used to screen for diabetes but this is not recommended because of the low sensitivity and poor specificity. In general the renal capacity to re-absorb glucose from the proximal tubule is only exceeded when the average glucose is greater than 11 mmol/l and therefore early diabetes will be missed if this test is employed. It may be considered when a patient refuses blood testing [21].

Cardiovascular Disease

Assessment of cardiovascular risk involves the measurement of age, gender, smoking, diabetes, blood pressure and fasting total and HDL cholesterol to calculate a score based on one of the risk engines [17]. Much of the clinical information is collected routinely and the measurement of total and HDL cholesterol involves a single blood test. Although the latter should ideally be obtained after a 10-hour fast, food has little impact on total or HDL cholesterol and therefore a non-fasting sample can be used to provide useful clinical information.

The distribution of test values in the target population should be known and a suitable cut-off level defined and agreed

Diabetes

The screening test employs the measurement of blood glucose and therefore may be diagnostic as well as a screening test. A diagnosis of diabetes is made when a fasting blood glucose value is greater than or equal to 7.0 mmol/l, or a random glucose, or 2-hour glucose during a glucose tolerance test is greater than 11 mmol/l. Glucose levels exhibit a skewed normal distribution within the population and the values that divide diabetes from normal are largely arbitrary. Historically, there has been considerable debate about the diagnostic glucose concentration, but currently there is an international consensus based on the levels that put an individual at risk of diabetic microvascular complications, in particular retinopathy [23].

Intermediate glucose abnormalities are also recognized: impaired fasting glycaemia reflects a fasting glucose between 6.0 and 7.0 mmol/l while impaired glucose tolerance refers to a 2-hour glucose of 7.8–11.0 mmol/l. Collectively, these two conditions have been referred to as 'pre-diabetes' because around 6–7% of these individuals will develop diabetes each year. In addition, these individuals are at increased risk of cardiovascular disease. There is less consensus about what constitutes an abnormal random glucose because of the variability of glucose following a meal. Nevertheless it would be reasonable to assume that those with a glucose greater than 7.0 mmol/l should undergo further investigation.

Cardiovascular Disease

Risk engines to assess the chance of a cardiovascular event over a 10-year period have been extensively studied and validated for the general population [17]. These risk engines may underestimate the risk of cardiovascular disease in people with SMI because the excess prevalence of CVD is not wholly explained by traditional risk factors raising the possibility that other unmeasured factors may be important in the aetiology of CVD in people with SMI [17]. As such, the current risk engines may lack sensitivity to detect people with SMI at high risk of CVD. There is no reason, however, to suggest that there is reduced specificity in this group and therefore if a high risk individual is identified, primary prevention should be instituted. Further research is needed to validate the current risk engines in people with SMI.

Although primary prevention trials have shown clinical effectiveness in people with a 10-year risk as low as 10%, there is less consensus about the risk threshold at which primary prevention is recommended. This is now largely an economic question as the number needed to treat to prevent one event increases as the absolute risk of an event decreases.

The test should be acceptable to the population

No research has been performed to determine the acceptability of diabetes and CVD disease screening in people with SMI. Our own experience would suggest that patient acceptability may be an issue. Locally, we have undertaken a study to evaluate the prevalence of diabetes and metabolic syndrome among people with schizophrenia and bipolar illness living in different settings. We have invited individuals to undergo physical health screening and have experienced suspicion and lack of consent from some people with SMI. This may reflect the nature of a research study and therefore physical health screening may be easier to undertake in routine clinical practice but this should not be assumed.

It is also important to assess the acceptability of physical health screening among health care professionals. In the UK, the National Institute of Health and Clinical Excellence (NICE) guidance is clear that the responsibility for physical health screening lies with primary care with secondary care taking responsibility for those patients who do not see the general practitioner [3]. This recommendation should ensure that all people with SMI receive the screening they need. In reality, we know from studies in the UK and elsewhere that screening is not taking place and there is a high prevalence of undiagnosed disease.

There should be an agreed policy on the further diagnostic investigation of individuals with a positive test result and on the choices available to those individuals

Diabetes

The screening test itself may be diagnostic for diabetes, but if the patient is asymptomatic, the diagnosis should be confirmed by a further test, as two blood samples are needed to diagnose diabetes in an asymptomatic individual. The WHO recommends that the confirmatory test should be a 75-gram oral glucose tolerance test. However, if the fasting blood glucose of the 75-gram OGTT confirms the diagnosis, it is unnecessary to complete the test.

Cardiovascular Disease

Once an individual is recognized as being at high risk of CVD, no further cardiovascular investigations are required unless the person has symptoms of CVD. Some treatment requires specific monitoring of other biochemical measures and therefore some additional investigation may be needed to ensure the safety of the medication. An example of this would be the assessment of liver function in those about to receive statins, or urea and electrolytes prior to ACE inhibitors. Specific investigations may be indicated to address individual clinical findings. For example, thyroid function should be assessed in those with hyperlipidaemia as undiagnosed hypothyroidism may lead to hypercholesterolaemia.

The Treatment

There should be an effective treatment or intervention for patients identified through early detection, with evidence of early treatment leading to better outcomes than late treatment

Diabetes

The United Kingdom Prospective Diabetes Study (UKPDS) has provided convincing evidence that improved glycaemic control reduces the incidence of microvascular complications. Individuals with newly diagnosed type 2 diabetes were randomized to received intensive or conventional hypoglycaemic management [24]. Over the median 10-year follow-up period, the HbA_{1c} was reduced by a mean of 0.9% in the intensive treatment group and this group experienced 25% fewer microvascular events.

Cardiovascular Disease

There are now many powerful clinical studies which confirm that primary prevention with lipid lowering drugs, aspirin, and antihypertensives, particularly inhibitors of the renin-angiotensin system, are associated with reductions in cardiovascular events [15].

There should be agreed evidence-based policies covering which individuals should be offered treatment and the appropriate treatment to be offered

Once a diagnosis of diabetes is made, all patients should be offered treatment for their diabetes. There are guidelines that determine the goals of treatment and well established algorithms that set out which treatments should be offered and when. Similarly for cardiovascular disease, there are targets for cholesterol reduction and blood pressure control and treatments. For both diabetes and CVD, however, there is debate about the precise targets. For example, for diabetes, the target glycosylated haemoglobin range between 6.0 and 7.5%. A further example is total cholesterol targets; the Joint British Societies recommend that the target total cholesterol should be 4 mmol/l [25] while the NSF for Cardiovascular Disease recommends 5 mmol/l, a figure echoed by the General Medical Services contract [15, 16].

Some of this debate reflects the date of publication of the guidance, which in turn reflects the available knowledge at that time and the effectiveness of treatment to achieve the target, but some may reflect financial restrictions within health care systems.

Clinical management of the condition and patient outcomes should be optimised in all health care providers prior to participation in a screening programme

Who provides what care is likely to be determined by health care setting. The many models of care prevent a detailed discussion of this criterion because what might be applicable in one country may not apply in another with a different health care model. UK government policy has encouraged a shift for the management of chronic illnesses from secondary care providers to primary care. The early management of diabetes and cardiovascular disease prevention falls within this remit and therefore most general practitioners have the necessary skills to undertake this care, with support from secondary care.

Although this criterion is fulfilled for the general population, and in theory the physical health care of those with SMI should be no different, there is less evidence that diabetes and cardiovascular disease management is optimal in people with SMI. Our local audit demonstrated a high prevalence of undiagnosed and untreated cardiovascular risk factors. There are several barriers that prevent high quality physical health care for those with SMI, including patient factors such as reluctance to comply with medication and system failures such as poor communication between primary and psychiatric care.

Further training on this topic, however, is probably needed for health care professionals working in mental health settings.

The Screening Programme

Currently there are no formalized screening programmes for diabetes and CVD risk factors in SMI and therefore most of the remaining criteria are not fulfilled, but nevertheless it is instructive to consider these to gain an understanding of what further research is needed to justify screening. Although some of these criteria are best applied to large national programmes, the principles are also important for locally implemented screening.

There should be evidence from high quality randomised controlled trials that the screening programme is effective in reducing mortality or morbidity

There have been no randomized controlled trials evaluating the effectiveness of screening for either diabetes or cardiovascular risk in people with SMI.

The complete screening programme should be clinically, socially and ethically acceptable to health professionals and the public

The disparities between the health outcomes of those with SMI and the general population have recently been highlighted and there is recognition that the current situation is unacceptable and measures should be introduced to minimize the differences. This has not, however, been formally assessed.

The benefit from the screening programme should outweigh the physical and psychological harm

Screening for diabetes and cardiovascular disease risk is simple and does not involve any physical harm. The potential for bruising or infection at the site of venepuncture is trivial.

The potential for psychological harm in people with SMI has not been determined. We have experienced suspicion when offering physical health screening and the very offer of a blood test may cause some distress. Most people with SMI and their carers, however, welcome the increased attention now being paid to their physical health.

The effect of being given a diagnosis of diabetes or high risk of cardiovascular disease has not been determined in people with SMI. While this may cause psychological harm, this must be put in the context of the physical harm caused by undiagnosed diabetes and cardiovascular disease. It seems likely that the psychological harm of discovering at a later date that someone has developed significant cardiovascular disease or diabetic complications, which may have been preventable, would be greater than the harm caused by the screening.

The screening programme should be cost effective

The cost of screening for diabetes and cardiovascular disease is low in most countries, where all the blood tests are performed routinely in hospital biochemistry laboratories. Similarly the measurement of blood pressure, weight and waist circumference is undertaken cheaply. There are costs involved with the management by health care professionals of any screening programme and there are additional treatment costs for those identified with diabetes or cardiovascular disease.

Most of the health costs involved in the management of either diabetes or cardiovascular disease relate to the treatment of complications of the diseases. Therefore if the screening programme leads to a reduction or delay in the incidence of complications, it is likely to be cost effective. Cost effectiveness has not been evaluated in people with SMI.

There should be a plan for managing and monitoring the screening programme and an agreed set of quality assurance standards

At present, there is no formal screening programme for screening for physical health problems in people with SMI and any screening is opportunistic.

Adequate staffing and facilities for testing, diagnosis, treatment and programme management should be available prior to the commencement of the screening programme

Most primary care physicians already have the facilities for testing, diagnosis and treatment of diabetes and cardiovascular disease. As people with SMI comprise about 2% of the whole population, the additional workload to introduce effective screening for diabetes and CVD should not be excessive.

There is a need for better liaison between primary care and mental health services to ensure that all people with mental illness receive appropriate screening and treatment and that this is not left to chance. It is likely that no one system will fit all clinical settings and therefore it is important that there are locally approved arrangements made to manage the screening.

All other options for managing the condition should have been considered (e.g. improving treatment, providing other services), to ensure that no more cost-effective intervention could be introduced or current interventions increased within the resources available

The current lack of screening for diabetes and cardiovascular is almost certainly leading to excess morbidity and mortality in those with SMI and it is unlikely that measures other than the ones proposed will be more cost effective in reducing this disease burden.

Evidence-based information, explaining the consequences of testing, investigation and treatment, should be made available to potential participants to assist them in making an informed choice

There is a wealth of information available for the general public to help them decide about screening for diabetes or CVD. Research is needed to assess the impact of this material in people with SMI. Both psychiatry and primary care physicians have a responsibility to ensure that people with mental illness are given the opportunity to make an informed choice about screening.

Public pressure for widening the eligibility criteria for reducing the screening interval, and for increasing the sensitivity of the testing process, should be anticipated. Decisions about these parameters should be scientifically justifiable to the public

Most recommendations for physical health screening in mental illness suggest an annual assessment. Given the natural history of both diabetes and cardiovascular disease, it is unlikely that there will be pressure to increase the frequency of this testing given the experience within the general population.

Table 4. Suggested screening protocol for diabetes and cardiovascular risk

	Test	Frequency
Diabetes	Fasting or random glucose	Before treatment initiation or switch 3–4 months later Annually thereafter
Cardiovascular disease	Lipid profile (ideally fasting)	Before treatment initiation or switch 3–4 months later Annually thereafter
	Blood pressure	Annual assessment
	Weight	Assess every visit. Weekly in the first 6 weeks of treatment
	Smoking	Assess every visit

Conclusion

The increased burden of physical illness and high rates of undiagnosed diabetes and cardiovascular disease provide a strong imperative to screen for these conditions in people with SMI (table 4). Most of the criteria relating to the illnesses and their screening tests are fulfilled. Although some of the criteria used to evaluate a screening programme are not satisfied, this is largely because formal screening has not yet taken place. There is a clear need to introduce screening for diabetes and CVD risk factors but at the same time, further research is needed to evaluate these interventions.

References

1 Brown S, Inskip H, Barraclough B: Causes of the excess mortality of schizophrenia. Br J Psychiatry 2000;177:212–217.

2 Osborn DP, Levy G, Nazareth I, Petersen I, Islam A, King MB: Relative risk of cardiovascular and cancer mortality in people with severe mental illness from the United Kingdom's General Practice Research Database. Arch Gen Psychiatry 2007;64:242–249.

3 National Institute for Clinical Excellence (NICE): Schizophrenia: core interventions in the treatment and management of schizophrenia in primary and secondary care. Clinical guidelines 1. London 2002; http://www.nice.org.uk. Accessed 18 March 08

4 'Schizophrenia and Diabetes 2003' Expert Consensus Meeting, Dublin, 3–4 October 2003: consensus summary. Br J Psychiatry 2004;47(suppl): 112–114.

5 Expert Group: Metabolic and lifestyle issues and severe mental illness: new connections to well-being. J Psychopharmacol 2005;19(suppl):118–122.

6 American Diabetes Association, American Psychiatric Association, American Association of Clinical Endocrinologists, North American Association for the Study of Obesity: Consensus development conference on antipsychotic drugs and obesity. Diabetes Care 2004;27:596–601.

7 Diabetes UK: Early identification of people with type 2 diabetes. http://www.diabetes.org.uk/Documents/Professionals/Earlyid_TYPE2_PS.doc.2006.Accessed 18 March 2008.

8 Marder SR, Essock SM, Miller AL, Buchanan RW, Casey DE, Davis JM, Kane JM, Lieberman JA, Schooler NR, Covell N, Stroup S, Weissman EM, Wirshing DA, Hall CS, Pogach L, Pi-Sunyer X, Bigger JT Jr, Friedman A, Kleinberg D, Yevich SJ, Davis B, Shon S: Physical health monitoring of patients with schizophrenia. Am J Psychiatry 2004; 161:1334–1349.

9 Canadian Diabetes Association: Clinical Practice Guidelines Expert Committee. CDA 2003 Clinical Practice Guidelines for the Prevention and Management of Diabetes: Screening and Prevention. Can J Diabetes 2003;27(suppl 2):10–13.
10 Lambert TJ, Chapman LH: Diabetes, psychotic disorders and antipsychotic therapy: a consensus statement. Med J Aust 2004;181:544–548.
11 UK National Screening Committee: Criteria for appraising the viability, effectiveness and appropriateness of a screening programme. http://www.nsc.nhs.uk/pdfs/criteria.pdf.2003. Accessed 17 March 2008.
12 Holt RI: Diagnosis, epidemiology and pathogenesis of diabetes mellitus: an update for psychiatrists. Br J Psychiatry Suppl 2004;47:55–63.
13 Audit Commission: Testing Times: A Review of Diabetes Services in England and Wales. London, Audit Commission, 2000.
14 Holt RI, Bushe C, Citrome L: Diabetes and schizophrenia 2005: are we any closer to understanding the link? J Psychopharmacol 2005;19(suppl):56–65.
15 Department of Health: National Service Framework for Coronary Heart Disease. London, Department of Health, 2000.
16 Department of Health: Investing in General Practice: The New General Medical Services Contract. London, Department of Health, 2003.
17 Grundy SM, Pasternak R, Greenland P, Smith S Jr, Fuster V: Assessment of cardiovascular risk by use of multiple-risk-factor assessment equations: a statement for healthcare professionals from the American Heart Association and the American College of Cardiology. Circulation 1999;100:1481–1492.
18 Tuomilehto J, Lindstrom J: The major diabetes prevention trials. Curr Diab Rep 2003;3:115–122.
19 Pendlebury J, Bushe CJ, Wildgust HJ, Holt RI: Long-term maintenance of weight loss in patients with severe mental illness through a behavioural treatment programme in the UK. Acta Psychiatr Scand 2007;115:286–294.
20 Anthonisen NR, Skeans MA, Wise RA, Manfreda J, Kanner RE, Connett JE: The effects of a smoking cessation intervention on 14.5-year mortality: a randomized clinical trial. Ann Intern Med 2005; 142:233–239.
21 Gough S, Peveler R: Diabetes and its prevention: pragmatic solutions for people with schizophrenia. Br J Psychiatry Suppl 2004;47 S106–S111.
22 van Winkel R, De Hert M, Van Eyck D, Hanssens L, Wampers M, Scheen A, Peuskens J, van Winkel R: Screening for diabetes and other metabolic abnormalities in patients with schizophrenia and schizoaffective disorder: evaluation of incidence and screening methods. J Clin Psychiatry 2006;67:1493–1500.
23 Report of the Expert Committee on the Diagnosis and Classification of Diabetes Mellitus. Diabetes Care 1997;20:1183–1197.
24 UK Prospective Diabetes Study (UKPDS) Group: Intensive blood-glucose control with sulphonylureas or insulin compared with conventional treatment and risk of complications in patients with type 2 diabetes (UKPDS 33). Lancet 1998;352:837–853.
25 JBS 2: Joint British Societies' guidelines on prevention of cardiovascular disease in clinical practice Heart 2005;91(suppl 5):v1–v52.

Prof. Richard Holt, MA, MB, BChir, PhD, FRCP, FHEA
IDS Building (MP887), Southampton General Hospital
Tremona Road
Southampton SO16 6YD (UK)
Tel. +44 23 8079 4665, Fax +44 23 8079 4945, E-Mail righ@soton.ac.uk

Thakore J, Leonard BE (eds): Metabolic Effects of Psychotropic Drugs.
Mod Trends Pharmacopsychiatry. Basel, Karger, 2009, vol 26, pp 82–89

Stress Axis Dysfunction: A Common Finding in Schizophrenia and the Metabolic Syndrome?

Natasha Afzal · Jogin Thakore

Neuroscience Centre, St. Vincent's Hospital Fairview, Dublin, Ireland

Abstract

Stress might be the unifying feature in both schizophrenia and the metabolic syndrome. It is possible that the perception of stress by those with schizophrenia is sufficiently altered so as to lead to a more frequent activation of the primary stress response, namely activation of the hypothalamic-pituitary-adrenal axis resulting in hypercortisolaemia. If so, this might lead to changes both in central (e.g. hippocampal function and structure) and peripheral effects (e.g. the adoption of a physical habitus characterized by upper body fat, insulin resistance/type 2 diabetes and ischaemic heart disease). Finally, 'switching off' of this stress axis may lead to reduction in both psychotic symptoms and metabolic derangements.

The metabolic syndrome (MetS) and illnesses that arise as a result of its presence are an integral part of schizophrenia. A debate still rages as to whether they are a consequence of certain neuroleptics that are commonly used in its treatment. Despite a huge increase in papers on the topic there is as such no definitive answer. What is clear is that many of these problems may be present before the onset of the illness (for example, in high-risk individuals) or before the commencement of treatment. An alternative explanation for the co-existence of schizophrenia and the physical states mentioned may be that they arise in parallel from a 'common soil'. A mediating factor for both may be dysfunction of the hypothalamic-pituitary-adrenal (HPA) axis.

This chapter aims to put forward evidence for this hypothesis. It will show how there is overactivity of the HPA axis in both schizophrenia and the MetS. The start of the chapter briefly outlines the normal function of the stress axis after which there is a description of how this endocrine system malfunctions in schizophrenia, both centrally and peripherally. Commonality between the physical manifestations of schizophrenia and Cushing's syndrome are enumerated. Finally, there is discussion about how stress may lead to the MetS and how pharmacological treatments for schizophrenia and MetS may work by effecting the HPA axis.

Hypothalamic-Pituitary-Adrenal Axis: Normal Physiology

From a physiological perspective, the response to stress is mediated by the HPA axis. A full description of this regulatory process is beyond the scope of this chapter and the reader is referred to Charmandari et al. [1] and Tsigos et al. [2] for a more comprehensive review. One of the primary mammalian responses to stress, be it psychological or physical, is activation of the HPA axis. In essence, the stressor stimulates the production and release of corticotropin-releasing hormone (CRH) from the paraventricular nucleus of the hypothalamus. CRH in turn causes the production and secretion of adrenocorticotropin hormone (ACTH) from the anterior pituitary gland. CRH is the prime secretagogue of ACTH though in situations of chronic stress this role is probably deferred to arginine vasopressin (AVP). ACTH travels to the adrenal glands where it stimulates the production and release of glucocorticoids (GC) such as cortisol. This series of hormonal releases occurs as a cascade and is termed the feedforward limb. As the HPA axis is a closed-loop system, cortisol acts to regulate its own secretion (feedback activity) by acting at a number of sites both peripherally (pituitary) and centrally (hypothalamus and hipppocampus). Cortisol acts on mineralocorticoid receptors (MR) and glucocorticoid receptors (GR) to maintain the circadian variation of the HPA axis. MRs are high-affinity receptors which are predominantly occupied under basal conditions and help maintain HPA axis tone, while GC, low-affinity receptors, are bound during times of stress and play a major role in 'switching off' the HPA axis. The hippocampus by virtue of the fact that it contains both MR and GR (the latter are also found in other areas of the CNS) plays a critical role in regulating HPA axis activity.

Hypothalamic-Pituitary-Adrenal Axis Dysfunction in Schizophrenia

A number of different groups measuring the HPA axis at rest have observed hypercortisolaemia and elevated ACTH levels in schizophrenia though this is not a universally reported finding [3–9]. There are probably a number of reasons why this is the case but the 3 most likely are differences in methodology, patients were receiving antipsychotic medication at the time of testing, or patients had been abruptly withdrawn from medications in order to produce a 'medication-free' scenario. Antipsychotics dampen activity of the HPA axis and such actions may occur via or independently of their actions on various monoaminergic systems [10]. Support that schizophrenia itself may be associated with increased HPA axis activity has come from endocrine and neuroimaging studies in drug-naïve first-episode patients (10% larger pituitary volume) and high-risk subjects (who showed a 20% increase of developing psychosis with each further 10% increase in pituitary size) [11].

Dynamic challenges of the HPA axis have also provided conflicting results probably for the same reasons quoted above. That aside, the dexamethasone suppression test (dexamethasone normally inhibits the secretion of ACTH and cortisol) is abnormal in nearly 50% of subjects with schizophrenia [12] though this is not a very sensitive test as such findings have also been shown in post-traumatic stress disorder [13] and Alzheimer's disease [14]. Delta-9-tetrahydro-cannbinol, an active cannabis ingredient, when given to subjects with schizophrenia results in high cortisol levels and can cause a heightening of positive, negative and cognitive symptoms [15]. ACTH increases are greater in patients than matched controls when metabolic stress is induced centrally by 2-deoxy-D-glucose (2-DG) [5] while some investigators have shown that CRH-stimulated ACTH and cortisol are normal; however, pretreatment with dexamethasone leads to increased cortisol secretion in patients with established schizophrenia [16].

Vasopressinergic function is altered in schizophrenia as is indicated by the higher than expected rates of syndrome of inappropriate antidiuretic hormone section [17, 18]. Furthermore, osmotic stimuli [19] resulted in patients secreting greater amounts of ACTH and cortisol despite secreting similar amounts of AVP, while Jansen and Gispen-de Wied [20] subjected patients to psychosocial and physical stressors but found that only the former resulted in a blunted cortisol response. Metoclopramide is unique in its ability to stimulate AVP release and does so without altering plasma intracellular glucose deprivation, osmolality, or peripheral haemodynamics [9, 21–24]. Walsh et al. [25] have shown that metoclopramide induced patients to secrete higher levels of ACTH and cortisol though AVP responses were similar in first-episode drug-naïve patients and their matched controls, a finding that may be explained by the fact that conditions of chronic stress increase pituitary responsiveness to AVP [26].

Altered stress responses in schizophrenia may have genetic underpinnings as is suggested by the findings that unaffected siblings of those with schizophrenia have exaggerated ACTH responses to stress [27], while Myin-Germeys et al. [28] have shown that those at high risk have increased behavioural sensitivity to daily life stressors. Brunelin et al. [29] have shown that 2-deoxyglucose induces a greater release of ACTH and homovanillic acid (a breakdown metabolite of dopamine and noradrenaline) in patients with schizophrenia with siblings have a response intermediate to probands and controls.

Lack of or poorly functioning GR can also lead to an overactive HPA axis and such changes have been seen in subjects with schizophrenia. i.e. GR mRNA numbers in the frontal cortices, amygdala and hippocampus (dentate gyrus, CA1, CA3 and CA4) [30, 31] although these changes also occur in other psychiatric illnesses such as bipolar disorder and major depression [32]. Further evidence of GR dysfunction may come from the observation that acutely administered dexamethasone leads to growth hormone release in healthy controls; a response dependent upon dexamethasone acting on GR located within the hypothalamus [33]. In schizophrenia, Thakore et al. [34] have shown that dexamethasone-induced growth hormone responses are blunted, indicating either a central reduction or dysfunction of GR.

Central and Physical Effects of Hypercortisolaemia

A well-established effect of high levels of cortisol is hippocampal shrinkage [35]. Compared to healthy controls both first-episode and patients with chronic schizophrenia have reduced hippocampal volumes as demonstrated by imaging and neuropathological studies [36, 37]. Such structural changes are associated with functional deficits in memory (verbal) and executive function [38]. The exact etiology of hippocampal volume reduction remains unclear but is attributed to both genetic and environmental factors such as, prenatal exposure to maternal stress, iatrogenic glucocorticoid administration, illicit drug usage and alcohol abuse and perinatal complications [39, 40].

Yet GCs also have peripheral effects as manifested by Cushing's disease (due to a pituitary basophil adenoma) or Cushing's syndrome (most commonly due to exogenous steroid administration) [41, 42]. GR are also located peripherally, for example in subcutaneous and visceral fat deposits, and it should come as no surprise that high levels of cortisol have peripheral effects such as increasing visceral fat deposits [43, 44]. Upper body fat, which consists of subcutaneous and visceral fat depots as is defined as a waist to hip ratio of 0.85 in women and 0.95 in men, is associated with greater metabolic disturbance than those with a predominantly lower fat distribution [45]. The exact mechanisms that underlie this process are still incompletely understood. However, we do know that obesity and free fatty acids (FFAs) in excess [46–49] leads to:

(1) Increases in glucose production, a decrease in peripheral glucose uptake, oxidation and storage which can lead to type 2 diabetes.
(2) Increases in insulin secretion and β-cell dysfunction which can lead to type 2 diabetes.
(3) Ischaemic heart disease either via hypertension or direct endothelial damage.

Chronic stress, in the form of elevated cortisol, can lead to a preferential increase in GR receptor density within visceral fat stores and an alteration in the activity of key enzymes which are known to reduce fat stores within the abdomen [50, 51].

These enzymes are:

(1) Lipoprotein lipase (LPL): LPL stimulates FFA uptake by the hydrolysis of meal-derived chylomicrons such as very-low-density lipoprotein and low-density lipoprotein at the level of the vascular endothelium. Thus released, FFAs can enter the adipocytes or the circulation directly.
(2) Hormone-sensitive lipase (HSL): This enzyme reduces adipocyte fat content.

Cortisol or GCs are known to increase the activity of LPL and reduce the activity of HSL thereby increasing the storage of upper body fat. Such intra-abdominal fat is associated with insulin resistance though the direction of causality is still open to debate. What is not doubted are the effects of such an adverse metabolic cocktail, namely, type 2 diabetes.

Stress, Obesity and Metabolic Syndrome

The perception and interpretation of stress determines the actual response any individual has to the stress presented [52]. A meta-analysis has shown that in addition to being activated when a physical threat is perceived, the HPA axis is also activated when there is a threat to one's social esteem and status [53]. In the context of schizophrenia, a misinterpretation of harmless environmental cues (psychological or physical) can be deemed a stressor and hence provoke a biological response.

So, can perceived stress and its biological correlate lead to metabolic disturbance? The answer would seem to be yes, in that, stress be it social or work-related leads to an immediate activation of the sympatho-adrenal network which leads to an outpouring of norepinephrine and cortisol which in healthy non-obese individuals results in tachycardia, a reflex vasodilation and the disposal of glucose while the opposite metabolic effects are seen in obesity [54]. The origin of the stress can be work-related or otherwise, as suggested in a study by Chandola et al. [55] who found that such stress was associated with higher cortisol levels in the morning and was directly related to the future development of IHD.

Healthy individuals respond to stress in a unitary fashion with the activation, as mentioned already, of the sympatho-adrenal system and the HPA axis resulting in an increase of cortisol and epinephrine. One immediate consequence of this is an increase in resting heart rate and a reduction of vascular resistance. In those individuals who are obese or have insulin resistance, endothelial dysfunction can dampen the compensatory reduction of blood pressure and limit glucose disposal in response to stress. These events can lead to central obesity and the development of certain features of the MetS.

From a cellular perspective, some investigators have suggested that the MetS may in fact be an intracellular manifestation of Cushing's syndrome [56, 57]. Evidence for this hypothesis has come primarily from examining the workings of 11β-hydroxysteroid dehydrogenase type 1 (11β-HSD1), which converts inactive cortisone to active cortisol. An in vitro study has found that fat-cell derived cytokines (e.g. IL-6 and TNF-α) acted in concert to increase the hepatocyte expression of 11β-HSD1, which increases the intracellular levels of cortisol. The same cytokines acted synergistically to increase the expression of GR receptors thereby potentiating the effects of an already readily available cortisol. The net effect would be to alter lipid and glucose metabolism, both key features of NetS. Furthermore, it would appear that commonly used anti-diabetic agents such as PPARγ/PPARα agonists, reduce the transcription of 11β-HSD1 leading to the question of whether agents that directly or indirect impact on the HPA axis can lead to an amelioration of symptoms associated with schizophrenia or indeed the MetS. In an elegant review of the stress-diathesis model of schizophrenia, Walker et al. [58] cite examples of how commonly used antipsychotics have a 'dampening' effect on the HPA axis which is associated with a reduction of psychotic symptoms adding further face validity to the hypothesis that stress dysfunction may play a central role in the pathogenesis of this serious mental illness.

In summary, stress may play an important mediator in both schizophrenia and the MetS. Activation of the HPA axis is a consequence of physical and psychological stressors, the latter including perceived threats to self-integrity and esteem. Dysfunction of the HPA axis occurs in both MetS and schizophrenia. Although cortisol is crucial for life, in excess can become the source of hippocampal shrinkage and visceral fat expansion, resulting in cognitive deficits and possibly insulin resistance. Preliminary evidence would suggest that restoration of normal HPA axis function by anti-diabetic agents in MetS or antipsychotics in schizophrenia may lead to an amelioration of physical or psychological symptoms.

References

1 Charmandari E, Kino T, Souvatzoglou E, Chrousos GP: Pediatric stress: hormonal mediators and human development. Horm Res 2003;59:161–179.
2 Tsigos C, Chrousos GP: Hypothalamic-pituitary-adrenal axis, neuroendocrine factors and stress. J Psychosom Res 2002;53:865–871.
3 Gil-Ad I, Dickerman, Z, Amdusky S, Laron Z: Diurnal rhythm of plasma beta endorphin, cortisol and growth hormone in schizophrenics as compared to control subjects. Psychopharmacology 1986;88:496–499.
4 Whalley LJ, Christie JE, Blackwood DH, Bennie J, Dick H, Blackburn IM, Fink G. Disturbed endocrine function in the psychoses. I. Disordered homeostasis or disease process? Br J Psychiatry 1989;155:455–461.
5 Brier A, Buchanan RW: The effects of metabolic stress on plasma progesterone in healthy volunteers and schizophrenic patients. Life Sci 1992;51:1527–1534.
6 Kaneda Y, Fujii A, Ohmori T: The hypothalamic-pituitary-adrenal axis in chronic schizophrenic patients long-term treated with neuroleptics. Prog Neuro-Psychopharmacol Biol Psychiatry 2002;26: 935–938.
7 Van Cauter, E, Linkowski P, Kerkhofs M, Hubain P, L'Hermite-Baleriaux M, Leclercq R, Brasseur M, Copinschi G, Mendelwicz J: Circadian and sleep-related endocrine rhythms in schizophrenia. Arch Gen Psychiatry 1991;48:348–356.
8 Rao M, Strebel B, Halaris A, Gross G, Braunig P, Marler M: Circadian rhythm of vital signs, norepinephrine, epinephrine, thyroid hormones and cortisol in schizophrenia. Psychiatry Res 1995;57: 21–39.
9 Elman I, Adler CM, Malhotra AK, Bir C, Pickar D, Breier A: Effect of acute metabolic stress on pituitary-adrenal axis activation in patients with schizophrenia. Am J Psychiatry 1998;155:979–981.
10 Meador-Woodruff JH, Greden JF: Effects of psychotropic medications on hypothalamic-pituitary-adrenal regulation. Neurol Clin 1988;6:225–234.
11 Pariante CM: Pituitary volume in psychosis: the first review of the evidence. J Psychopharmacol 2008;22(2 suppl):76–81.
12 Sharma R, Pandey G, Janicak P, et al: The effect of diagnosis and age on the DST: a meta-analytic approach. Biol Psychiatry 1993;24:555–568.
13 Yehuda R, Southwick S, Nussbaum G, et al: Low urinary cortisol excretion in patients with posttraumatic stress disorder. J Nerv Ment Dis 1990;178: 366–369.
14 de Leon M, McRae T, Tsai J, et al: Abnormal cortisol response in Alzheimer's disease linked to hippocampal atrophy. Lancet 1988;ii:391–92.
15 D'Souza DC, Abi-Saab WM, Madonick S, et al: Delta-9-tetrahydrocannabinol effects in schizophrenia: implications for cognition, psychosis, and addiction. Biol Psychiatry 2005;57:594–608.

16 Lammers C, Garcia Boreguero D, Schmider J, et al: Combined dexamethasone/corticotrophin releasing hormone test in patients with schizophrenia and in normal controls. Biol Psychiatry 1995;38:803–807.

17 Goldman MB, Blake K, Marks RC, Hedeker D, Luchins DJ: Association of nonsuppression on the DST with primary polydipsia in chronic schizophrenia. Am J Psychiatry 1993;150:653–655.

18 Goldman MB, Robertson GL, Luchins DJ, Hedeker P, Pandey GN: Psychotic exacerbations and enhanced vasopressin secretion in schizophrenic patients with hyponatremia and polydipsia. Arch Gen Psychiatry 1997;54:443–449.

19 Hundt W, Kellner M, Wiedemann K: Neuroendocrine effects of a short-term osmotic stimulus in patients with chronic schizophrenia. World J Biol Psychiatry 2001;2:27–33.

20 Jansen LMC, Gispen-de Wied CC, Kahn RS: Selective impairments in the stress response in schizophrenic patients. Psychopharmacology 2000; 149:319–325.

21 Kendler KS, Weitzman RE, Rubin R: Lack of arginine vasopressin response to central dopamine blockade in normal adults. J Clin Endocrinol Metab 1978; 47:204–207.

22 Nomura K, Kurimoto F, Demura H, Sakurai,H, Nomura T, Zibiki K, Naruse M, Kanai N, Shizume K: The effects of metoclopramide on plasma vasopressin in man. Clinical Endocrinol 1984;21:117–121.

23 Norbiato G, Bevilacqua M, Chebat E, Bertora P, Cavaiani P, Baruto C, Fumagalli S, Raggi U: Metoclopramide increases vasopressin secretion. J Clin Endocrinol Metab 1986;63:747–750.

24 Seki K, Kato T, Sekiya S: Corticotrophin and vasopressin responses to metoclopramide in patients with hypothalamic amenorrhoea. Clin Endocrinol 1997;46:203–207.

25 Walsh P, Spelman L, Sharifi N, Thakore JH: Male patients with paranoid schizophrenia have greater ACTH and cortisol secretion in response to metoclopramide-induced AVP release. Psychoneuroendocrinology 2005;30:431–437.

26 Rabadan-Diehl C, Aguilera G: Glucocorticoids increase vasopressin V1b receptor coupling to phospholipase C. Endocrinology 1998;139:3220–3226.

27 Marcelis M, Cavalier E, Gielen J, Delespaul P, Van Os J: Abnormal response to metabolic stress in schizophrenia: marker of vulnerability or acquired sensitization? Psychol Med 2004;34:1103–1111.

28 Myin-Germeys I, Marcelis M, Krabbendam L, Delespaul P, van Os J: Subtle fluctuations in psychotic phenomena as functional states of abnormal dopamine reactivity in individuals at risk. Biol Psychiatry 2005;58:105–110.

29 Brunelin J, d'Amato T, Van OS J, Dalery J, Suaud-Chagny MF, Saoud M: Serotonergic response to stress: a protective factor against abnormal dopaminergic reactivity in schizophrenia? Eur Psychiatr 2007;22:362–364.

30 Perlman WR, Webster MJ, Kleinman JK, Weickert CS: Reduced glucocorticoid and estrogen receptor messenger ribonucleic acid levels in the amygdala of patients with major mental illness. Biol Psychiatry 2004;56:844–852.

31 Xing GQ, Russell S, Webster MJ, Post RM: Decreased expression of mineralocorticoid receptor mRNA in the prefrontal cortex in schizophrenia and bipolar disorder. Int J Neuropsychopharmacol 2004;7:143–153.

32 Webster M, O'Grady J, Orthmann C, et al: Decreased glucocorticoid receptor mRNA levels in individuals with depression, bipolar disorder and schizophrenia. Schizophrenia Res 2000;41:111.

33 Thakore JH, Dinan TG: Growth hormone secretion: the role of glucocorticoids. Life Sci 1994;14:1083–1099.

34 Thakore JH, Dinan TG: Are blunted dexamethasone-induced growth hormone responses specific for depression? Psychol Med 1996;26:1053–1059.

35 Sapolsky RM. Stress and plasticity in the limbic system. Neurochem Res 2003;28:1735–1742.

36 Geuze E, Vermetten E, Bremner JD: MR-based in vivo hippocampal volumetrics: 2. Findings in neuropsychiatric disorders. Mol Psychiatry 2005;10: 160–184.

37 Steen RG, Mull C, McClure R, Hamer RM, Lieberman JA: Brain volume in first-episode schizophrenia: systematic review and meta-analysis of magnetic resonance imaging studies. Br J Psychiatry 2006;188:510–518.

38 Antonova E, Sharma T, Morris R, Kumari V: The relationship between brain structure and neurocognition in schizophrenia: a selective review. Schizophr Res 2004;70:117–145.

39 McNeil TF, Cantor-Graae E, Weinberger DR: Relationship of obstetric complications and differences in size of brain structures in monozygotic twin pairs discordant for schizophrenia. Am J Psychiatry 2000;157:203–212.

40 van Erp TG, Saleh PA, Huttunen M, et al. Hippocampal volumes in schizophrenic twins. Arch Gen Psychiatry 2004;61:346–353.

41 Meador CK, Liddle GW, Island DP, et al: Cause of 'Cushing's syndrome' in patients with tumors arising from non-endocrine tissue. J Clin Endocrinol Metab 1962;22:693–703.

42 Orth DN: Ectopic hormone production; in Felig P, Baxter JD, Broadus AE, et al (eds): Endocrinology and Metabolism, ed 2. New York, McGraw-Hill, 1987, pp 1692–1735.

43 Rebuffe-Scrive M, Lundholm K, Bjorntorp P: Glucocorticoid binding of human adipose tissue. Eur J Clin Invest 1985;15:267–272.
44 Pedersen SB, Jonier M, Richelsen B: Characterisation of regional and gender differences in glucocorticoid receptors and lipoprotein lipase activity in human adipose tissue. J Clin Endocrinol Metab 1994;78: 1354–1359.
45 Santosa S, Jensen MD: Why are we shaped differently and why does it matter? Am J Physiol 2008; 295:E531–E353.
46 Paolisso G, Tataranni PA, Foley JE, Bogardus C, Howard BV, Ravussin E: A high concentration of fasting plasma non-esterified fatty acids is a risk factor for the development of NIDDM. Diabetologia 1995;38:1213–1217.
47 Piro S, Spampinato D, Spadaro L, Oliveri CE, Purrello F, Rabuazzo AM: Direct apoptotic effects of free fatty acids on human endothelial cells. Nutr Metab Cardiovasc Dis 2008;18:96–104.
48 Pirro M, Mauriege P, Tchernof A, Cantin B, Dagenais GR, Despres JP, Lamarche B: Plasma free fatty acid levels and the risk of ischemic heart disease in men: prospective results from the Quebec Cardiovascular Study. Atherosclerosis 2002;160:377–384.
49 Prentki M: New insights into pancreatic beta-cell metabolic signaling in insulin secretion. Eur J Endocrinol 1996;134:272–286.
50 Bjorntorp P: The regulation of adipose tissue distribution in humans. Int J Obes 1996;20:291–302.
51 Ottoson M, Vikman-Adolfson K, Enerback S, Olivecrona G, Bjorntorp P: The effects of cortisol on the regulation of lipoprotein lipase activity in human adipose tissue. J Clin Endocrinol Metab 1994;79:820–825.
52 Lupien SJ: Stress and schizophrenia: the importance of cognition. Biol Psychiatry 2000;48:1119–1120.
53 Dickerson SS, Kemeny ME: Acute stressors and cortisol responses: a theoretical integration and synthesis of laboratory research. Psychol Bull 2004;130: 355–391.
54 Seematter G, Binnert C, Tappy L: Stress and metabolism. Metab Syndr Relat Disord 2005 3:8–13.
55 Chandola T, Britton A, Brunner E, Hemingway H, Malik M, Kumari M, Badrick E, Kivimaki M, Marmot M: Work stress and coronary heart disease: what are the mechanisms? Eur Heart J 2008;29:640–648.
56 Syed AA, Redfern CP, Weaver JU: In vivo and in vitro glucocorticoid sensitivity in obese people with cushingoid appearance. Obesity (Silver Spring) 2008;16:2374–2378.
57 Iwasaki Y, Takayasu S, Nishiyama M, Tsugita M, Taguchi T, Asai M, Yoshida M, Kambayashi M, Hashimoto K: Is the metabolic syndrome an intracellular Cushing state? Effects of multiple humoral factors on the transcriptional activity of the hepatic glucocorticoid-activating enzyme (11beta-hydroxysteroid dehydrogenase type 1) gene. Mol Cell Endocrinol 2008;285:10–18.
58 Walker E, Mittal V, Tessners K: Stress and the hypothalamic pituitary adrenal axis in the developmental course of schizophrenia. Annu Rev Clin Psychol 2008;4:189–216.

Jogin Thakore, MD, PhD, MRCPsych
Neuroscience Centre, St. Vincent's Hospital Fairview
Richmond Road
Dublin (Ireland)
Tel. +353 1 8842400, Fax +353 1 8370801,E-Mail jthakore@rcsi.ie

Thakore J, Leonard BE (eds): Metabolic Effects of Psychotropic Drugs.
Mod Trends Pharmacopsychiatry. Basel, Karger, 2009, vol 26, pp 90–104

Metabolic Syndrome in Psychiatric Inpatients Treated for Depression

John W. Goethe[a] · Bonnie L. Szarek[a] · Charles F. Caley[a,b]

[a]Burlingame Center for Psychiatric Research and Education, Institute of Living, Hartford, Conn., and
[b]University of Connecticut School of Pharmacy, Storrs, Conn., USA

Abstract

That metabolic syndrome (MetS) is associated with schizophrenia is well established but recent findings suggest that the risk of MetS may be similar in patients with major depressive disorder (MDD). The investigators identified all admissions age 18–59 with a clinical diagnosis of MDD (n = 1,776) at an urban, not-for-profit hospital in the US to determine the prevalence of MetS and of each of its five ATP III criteria. Descriptive statistics were used to determine the prevalence of MetS and its component measures and χ^2 analyses to compare these results with the most recent National Health and Nutrition Examination Survey Data (NHANES). Stepwise logistic regressions were used to identify associated demographic and clinical features. In the subset of patients for whom all metabolic measures were available (n = 1,028), 23.4% (n = 241) had MetS and 75.6% (n = 777) met at least one criterion for the syndrome. Compared with the NHANES sample, MDD patients were more likely to have elevated glucose ($p < 0.001$), decreased HDL cholesterol ($p < 0.001$), at least one ATP-III criterion present ($p < 0.001$), and the full syndrome (i.e. at least three ATP-III criteria) ($p = 0.003$). In the logistic regressions atypical antipsychotics were not associated with either an increased risk for MetS or the presence of ≥1 of the criteria. However, patients receiving venlafaxine were 65% more likely to have ≥1 criterion, and those receiving two or more antidepressants or an anticonvulsant were more likely to have the full syndrome (100% and 58% increased risk, respectively). Risk for MetS was more than doubled in patients ≥40 years, Latino females, and those with a co-diagnosis of borderline personality disorder.

Introduction

Background

Early studies of metabolic syndrome (MetS) in psychiatric patients found a higher than expected prevalence of this condition and found that it was associated with a diagnosis of schizophrenia and with exposure to atypical antipsychotics [1]. Only recently have investigators reported a similar prevalence in patients with major depressive disorder

(MDD). For example, in one study of outpatients with MDD the prevalence of MetS was 36% [2], which can be compared to a prevalence of 40.9% in outpatients with schizophrenia [3] and 26.7% in the US general population [4]. Findings from several other studies are similar [2, 5–11], but comparisons and conclusions are complicated by the lack of consensus about the optimal definition of MetS [12, 13]. An association between MetS and MDD is of interest for several reasons. Depression is far more common than schizophrenia, and any therapeutic or etiologic implications about MetS and MDD would be relevant for a large number of current patients as well as for individuals in the general population who may become depressed. Because MDD samples can be divided into subgroups based on pharmacotherapy (e.g. antidepressant monotherapy, polytherapy, use of antipsychotics), studies of depressed patients can assess the relative contributions to MetS of a number of psychotropics, not just the antipsychotics. In addition, the association between MetS and depression may be bi-directional. For example, in a study of nondepressed individuals, those with MetS at baseline were twice as likely as those without MetS to have depressive symptoms at follow up (OR = 2.1, 95% CI 1.2–3.8) [10]; in a study of patients with MDD, the prevalence of MetS was 57.9% in those who remained depressed 6 years after enrollment compared to 32.4% in those who were no longer depressed ($p = 0.034$) [2].

This Paper

Additional studies of MetS and depression are needed. There are few studies of MetS in severely depressed patients and little data about the potential contribution to MetS of the medications most commonly used to treat MDD. The authors present the results of a study of MetS in a large sample of inpatients being treated for MDD. They report the prevalence of MetS and the demographic, clinical, and treatment variables associated with increased risk for this syndrome. They also discuss the implications of these data for clinical practice.

Methods

Defining Metabolic Syndrome

There are different definitions of MetS, the most commonly referenced of which are those proposed by the National Cholesterol Education Program Adult Treatment Panel III (ATP-III), European Group for the Study of Insulin Resistance (EGIR), International Diabetes Federation Epidemiology Task Force Consensus Group (IDF), American Heart Association/National Heart, Lung, and Blood Institute (AHA/NHLBI), World Health Organization (WHO), and the American Association of Clinical Endocrinologists (AACE) [12, 14–18]. All include assessment of body fat, dyslipidemia, blood pressure, and glucose dysregulation, but different metrics and cutoffs are used. The most common measures of body fat are waist circumference (ATP-III, EGIR, IDF, AHA/NHLBI) and BMI (WHO, AACE) [12, 14–18]. Dyslipidemia measures include triglycerides (≥150 mg/dl) and HDL cholesterol (various cutoffs). In some definitions the blood pressure criterion is based on a measured diastolic and systolic reading at assessment (cutoffs vary), but in others (EGIR, IDF, AHA/NHLBI) proxies for elevated blood pressure such as receiving medication for hypertension are included. All definitions of MetS include impaired fasting glucose (FBS ≥100 or ≥110) as a criterion of glucose dysregulation, but two also use impaired glucose tolerance (WHO, EGIR), one includes receiving medication for elevated glucose (AHA/NHLBI), three include a diagnosis of diabetes mellitus (DM) (WHO, ATP-III, IDF), and two exclude patients with this diagnosis (EGIR, AACE); one definition also includes decreased insulin sensitivity (WHO), one (EGIR) includes plasma insulin >75th percentile, and two (WHO, AACE) include microalbuminuria and other features of insulin resistance.

For this study, the ATP III definition of MetS was used [14]. It requires the presence of at least three of five specified criteria: FBS ≥110 mg/dl, waist circumference (WC) >102 cm for men or >88 cm for women, blood pressure (BP) ≥130 mg Hg systolic/≥85 mg Hg diastolic, triglycerides ≥150 mg dl, and high-density lipoprotein cholesterol (HDL) <40 mg/dl for men or <50 mg/dl for women. Diagnosis of hypertension was substituted for blood pressure ≥130/85 because BP was not always recorded.

Procedures

This study was conducted at an urban, not-for-profit hospital between April 2005 and September 2007. Following IRB approval the investigators identified all admissions age 18–59 years with a clinical diagnosis of MDD (n = 1,776). To determine the prevalence of MetS and of each of its component measures, the following information was collected: BMI, WC, triglycerides and HDL levels, FBS, diagnosis of hypertension (HTN) or DM, and receiving medication for DM or dyslipidemia.

Statistics

Descriptive statistics were used to determine the prevalence of MetS and its component measures; χ^2 analyses were used to compare these results with the most recent National Health and Nutrition Examination Survey Data (NHANES) [19]. Because there are associations between the MetS criteria [20], we used the Mantel-Haenszel Common Odds Ratio Estimate (95% CI) to determine the strength of association between all possible pairings of the ATP III criteria. Stepwise logistic regressions were used to identify variables associated with the presence of each of the following dependent variables: ≥3 ATP-III criteria (i.e. MetS), ≥1 ATP-III criterion, WC criterion, BMI >30, FBS criterion, triglycerides criterion, HDL criterion, diagnosis of HTN, DM, or dyslipidemia, receiving medication for DM or dyslipidemia, FBS >110 and/or DM diagnosis and/or on DM medication, increased triglycerides and/or decreased HDL cholesterol and/or diagnosis or medication for dyslipidemia. Independent variables for these analyses were: age ≥40, female, black, Latino (comparator is white), black female, black male, Latino female, Latino male, white female (comparator is white male), substance abuse/dependence, alcohol abuse/dependence, drug abuse/dependence, opioid dependence, cocaine dependence, psychotic depression, personality disorder, borderline personality disorder, prescribed antipsychotic, typical antipsychotic, atypical antipsychotic, aripiprazole, olanzapine, quetiapine, risperidone, ziprasidone, mirtazapine, venlafaxine, TCA, topiramate, valproate, lithium, clozapine or olanzapine, quetiapine or risperidone, aripiprazole or ziprasidone, H1 blockade (i.e. receiving clozapine, olanzapine, quetiapine, mirtazapine, TCA, or typical antipsychotic), 5HT2C blockade (i.e. receiving olanzapine, mirtazapine), >1 antidepressant, and >1 antipsychotic. OR with 95% CI are reported. The H1 and HT2C variables were added because both have been implicated in weight gain [17, 21–24].

Stepwise logistic regression was also used to identify any between-group differences in patients who had all ATP III measures recorded vs. those with one or more missing criteria. Independent variables in these analyses were: age ≥40 (utilized because 40 was the median age), female, black, Latino (white as comparator), substance abuse/dependence, alcohol abuse/dependence, drug abuse/dependence, psychotic depression, antipsychotic, and atypical antipsychotic.

FBS was documented for 96.6% of subjects, and for approximately three-quarters of the sample WC, triglycerides, and HDL were available (78.0, 71.6 and 71.3%, respectively). Missing data (e.g. due to invalid values, patient refusal) resulted in the creation of several subsamples. For example, all five ATP III measures were available on a subset of 1,028 patients (57.9% of the sample), and from this subset the prevalence of MetS was calculated. The prevalence of each individual measure is reported for the subset of subjects having a given criterion recorded: n = 1,386 (78.0%) for WC, n = 1,715 (96.6%) for FBS, n = 1,271 (71.6%) for triglycerides, n = 1,267 (71.3%) for HDL cholesterol. All subsamples were compared to the remainder of the sample to identify potential sample bias.

Sample

The sample as a whole (n = 1,776) had 1,096 (61.7%) females and 680 males; more than half were white (63.0%, n = 1119), 25.6% (n = 455) were Latino, and 11.4% (n = 202) were black. Mean age was 38.3 years (SD 11.3). The majority of patients (91.9%, n = 1,633) had recurrent depression; 36.4% (n = 646) had psychotic features. An Axis I co-diagnosis was present in 70.2% (n = 1246), and the most common was substance abuse/dependence (57.1%, 1014); 48.3% (n = 857) had a personality disorder, and the most common were personality disorder NOS (26.3%, n = 471) and borderline (15.4%, n = 274).

The subset of patients with all ATP III criteria recorded were more likely to be ≥40 years of age (OR = 1.36, CI 1.13–1.65) and to be on atypical antipsychotics (OR = 1.34, CI 1.10–1.63) but less likely to have a diagnosis of alcohol abuse/dependence (OR = 0.73, CI 0.60–0.89). Adding BMI and WC as independent variables revealed that the subset of patients who had triglycerides assessed were more likely to be ≥40 years of age (OR = 1.64, CI 1.27–2.12) and to meet the WC criterion (OR = 1.34, CI 1.04–1.63) but less likely to have a diagnosis of alcohol abuse/dependence (OR = 0.57, CI 0.44–0.74). Almost all patients in this subset (99.6%) also had HDL assessed.

Results

Pharmacotherapy

The pharmacotherapy for the sample is summarized in table 1. Almost all patients received an antidepressant (98.4%, n = 1747), most commonly an SSRI (70.3%, n = 1,248). The second most commonly used antidepressant was trazodone (21.2%, n = 377), but it was almost always given at bedtime in low dosages (50–150 mg) and was never used as monotherapy. A combination of antidepressants was given to 16.9% (n = 300) of the sample. Antipsychotics were prescribed for 58.3% of patients; 65 individuals were given a typical antipsychotic, but most of this subgroup (n = 44, 56.7%) also received an atypical agent. Among the atypicals prescribed, olanzapine and clozapine (those most implicated in MetS) [25, 26] were given to only 5.3% of patients (n = 94). An anticonvulsant was prescribed for 23.6% of patients (n = 419), and the most

Table 1. Pharmacotherapy for the sample

Psychotropic	n (%) receiving[1]
Antidepressant	1,747 (98.4)
Antipsychotic	1,035 (58.3)
Anticonvulsant	419 (23.6)
Lithium	40 (2.3)
Benzodiazepine	608 (34.2)

[1]Total >100% because many patients received >1 drug; 44% (n = 783) received 2, 26.0% (n = 462) received 3, 7.2% (n = 127) received ≥4.

commonly used were gabapentin (n = 192, 10.8%), lamotrigine (n = 85, 4.8%), and valproic acid (n = 81, 4.6%).

Prevalence of MetS

Table 2 displays the proportion of patients meeting each MetS criterion and compares these values with those for the general US population in the same age range (18–59 years) [19].

The prevalence found for the full syndrome (23.4%) and for the presence of at least one criterion (75.6%) were calculated for the subset of patients for whom all metabolic measures were available (n = 1,028). Among all patients studied, 14.9% (n = 264) had MetS and for 63.6% (n = 1,128) at least one criterion was present.

Compared with the NHANES sample, MDD patients were more likely to have elevated glucose ($\chi^2 = 12.18$, $p < 0.001$), decreased HDL cholesterol ($\chi^2 = 41.21$, $p < 0.001$), at least one ATP III criterion present ($\chi^2 = 12.32$, $p < 0.001$), and MetS (i.e., at least three ATP-III criteria) ($\chi^2 = 8.69$, $p = 0.003$). MDD patients were less likely than the NHANES sample to meet the hypertension criterion ($\chi^2 = 26.69$, $p < 0.001$), but in this study a recorded HTN diagnosis was substituted for the ATP III BP criterion used in NHANES.

Treatment and Demographic Variables Associated with MetS

In the logistic regressions atypical antipsychotics were not associated with either an increased risk for MetS or the presence of one or more of the five criteria (table 3). Psychotropic exposure was relevant, however. Patients receiving venlafaxine were 65% more likely to have ≥1 criteria, and those receiving two or more antidepressants

Table 2. Prevalence of MetS criteria: study sample vs. general population

Criterion	Study sample 4/05–9/07 n (%)	NHANES [19] 2003–2004 n (%)
WC (M >102 cm, F >88 cm)	671 (48.4)	1,583 (45.6)
FBS ≥110 mg/dl[c]	246 (14.3)	167 (10.4)
Triglycerides ≥150 mg/dl	409 (32.2)	480 (30.0)
HDL cholesterol*	465 (36.6)	901 (27.0)
Dx hypertension* (M <40 mg/dl, F <50 mg/dl)	298 (16.8)	682 (23.1)
≥1 ATP-III criterion*	777 (75.6)	897 (69.0)
≥3 ATP-III criteria*	241 (23.4)	240 (18.5)

Percent displayed is percent of the subgroup for whom measure(s) were available.
*Significant differences between MDD and NHANES ($p < 0.001$–0.003).

or an anticonvulsant were more likely to have the full syndrome (100 and 58% increased risk, respectively). Risk for MetS was more than doubled by three non-treatment variables: age ≥40, Latina female, and co-diagnosis of borderline personality disorder.

The associations between the independent variables and the individual components of MetS varied widely. The likelihood that the WC criterion was met was much greater for patients receiving two or more antipsychotics (OR = 2.44, CI 1.06–5.62), those taking more than one antidepressant (OR = 1.91, CI 1.40–2.62), those on aripiprazole or ziprasidone (OR = 1.62, CI 1.08–2.43), females (OR = 4.49, CI 3.30–6 11), and patients ≥40 years of age (OR = 1.76, CI 1.40–2.21). Triglycerides ≥150 mg/dl was associated with taking venlafaxine (OR = 1.46, CI 1.06–1.99), tricyclic antidepressants (OR = 2.11, CI 1.13–3.96), or an anticonvulsant (OR = 1.50, CI 1.14–1.98), as well as with age ≥40 years (OR = 1.69, CI 1.32–2.16) and with having a co-diagnosis of borderline personality disorder (OR = 1.65, CI 1.17–2.32). The individuals at increased risk on the HDL measure were those taking an anticonvulsant (OR = 1.45, CI 1.10–1.91) and black and Latino females (OR = 4.85, CI 2.15–10.91 and OR = 2.39, CI 1.75–3.29, respectively). On the FBS measure, high-risk patients were those ≥40 years of age (OR = 2.85, CI 2.12–3.82), Latino males (OR = 1.73, CI 1.15 = 3.63), and patients with a co-diagnosis of borderline personality disorder (OR = 1.84, CI 1.24–2.73). There were increased risks on the BP criterion for patients taking typical antipsychotics (OR = 2.07, CI 1.06–4.06) or ≥1 antidepressant (OR = 1.76, CI 1.26–2.46) and for those ≥40 years of age (OR = 6.81, CI 4.02–9.41). Of the variables

Table 3. Variables associated with increased risk of MetS

Independent variable	MetS[1] (n =1,028)[2] OR (CI)	≥1 criterion[3] (n = 1,028)[2] OR (CI)
Venlafaxine	–	1.65 (1.06–2.58)
>1 antidepressant	2.00 (1.25–2.95)	1.59 (1.04–2.42)
Anticonvulsant	1.58 (1.13–2.21)	–
Age ≥40	2.68 (1.94–3.70)	1.98 (1.46–2.68)
Black female	–	2.59 (1.28–5.26)
Latino female	2.18 (1.47–3.24)	2.48 (1.52–4.06)
Psychotic depression	–	1.79 (1.25–2.56)
Borderline personality disorder	2.19 (1.48–3.25)	1.78 (1.13–2.79)

[1]MetS = Metabolic syndrome (≥3 ATP III criteria present).
[2]Limited to those with all 5 ATP III measures.
[3]≥1 of the 5 ATP III criteria.

examined, age ≥40 years was associated with increased risk on the greatest number of MetS criteria: WC, triglycerides, FBS, and BP. 5HTC2 blockade drugs were associated with decreased risk on the WC measure (OR = 0.51, CI 0.35–0.72). Patients on H1 blockade drugs were less likely to have a diagnosis of HTN (OR = 0.64, CI 0.47–0.85), to have DM and/or to be taking DM medication (OR = 0.52, CI 0.32–0.83), to meet the triglyceride or HDL measures, or to have a diagnosis of dyslipidemia and/or a current order for a statin (OR = 1.42, CI 1.15–1.75). There were no other associations with 5HT2C or H1 blockade.

Figure 1 displays the prevalence of each MetS measure by race/gender. The WC and HDL criteria were more commonly met in black and Latina females and the triglyceride measure was more common in black females. Figure 2 shows the incremental increase in risk for Latina females relative to other subgroups in both prevalence of MetS and the presence of one or more of the criteria.

As expected there were associations between the five MetS measures. Only the HDL – FBS and HDL – BP associations were not statistically significant (OR = 1.25, CI 0.91–1.70, and OR = 1.11, CI 0.83–1.49, respectively). In all other instances the presence of any criterion was associated with an increased likelihood that any of the remaining criteria would also be present. Odds ratios varied from 1.64 (CI 1.35–2.89) for the WC-FBS association to 4.04 (CI 3.00–5.45) for the FBS-BP association. WC was highly associated with the BP criterion (OR = 3.13, CI 2.31–4.24) and with the two lipid measures (triglycerides: OR = 2.74, CI 2.09–3.60 and HDL: OR = 2.17, CI 1.67–2.81).

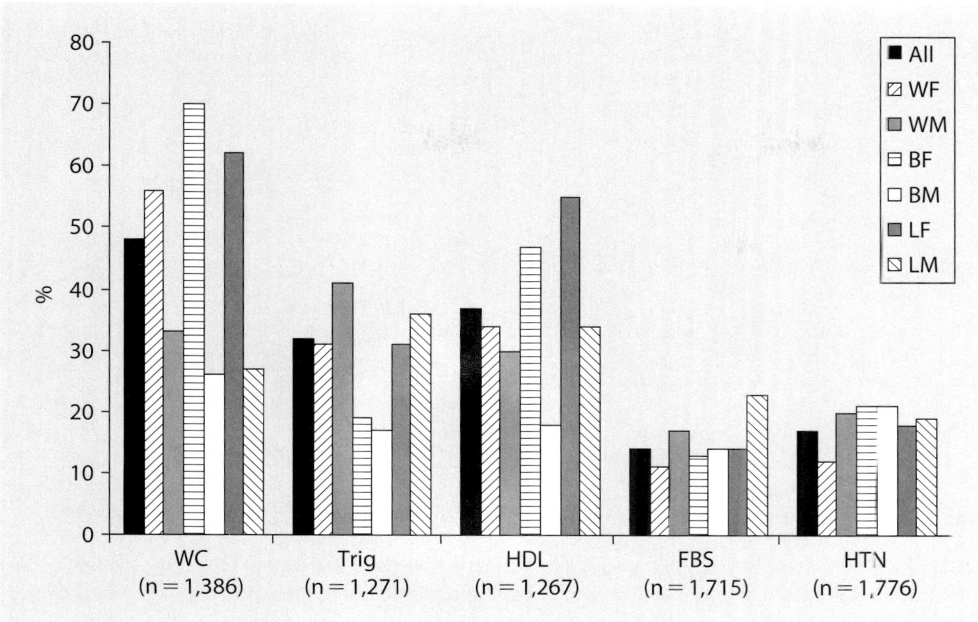

Fig. 1. Prevalence of each MetS criterion by race/gender. WF = White female, WM = white male, BF = black female, BM = black male, LF = Latina female, LM = Latino male, WC = waist circumference >102 cm for men or >88 cm for women, Trig = triglycerides ≥150 mg/dl, HDL cholesterol <40 mg/dl for men or <50 mg/dl for women, FBS = fasting blood sugar ≥110 mg/dl, HTN = hypertension diagnosis.

Effect of Using Other Definitions of MetS

Using other definitions for MetS would alter some of the findings reported above. For example, while 48.4% of the sample satisfied the ATP III criterion for body weight [27], only 28.0% met the World Health Organization criterion (BMI >30) [17]. Of patients with both WC and BMI recorded, nearly all at the BMI cut point (92.1%) met the WC criterion, but only 53.0% of those above the ATP III WC cut point had BMI >30. Comparing glycemic control measures, 14.3% had a FBS ≥110 but 19.3% were in 'dyscontrol' using as the criterion FBS ≥110 and/or a documented DM diagnosis and/or receiving a DM medication. The ATP III criteria for triglycerides and HDL were present in 32.2% and 36.6%, respectively, but 43.8% of the sample had one or both one of these measures and/or a diagnosis of dyslipidemia and/or receiving a statin.

Recognition of MetS in Clinical Practice

Some findings point to the possible under recognition and/or under treatment of metabolic dysfunction. For almost all patients without a DM diagnosis, FBS was <110 (90.2%, n = 1,379 of the 1,529 patients without a DM diagnosis and not

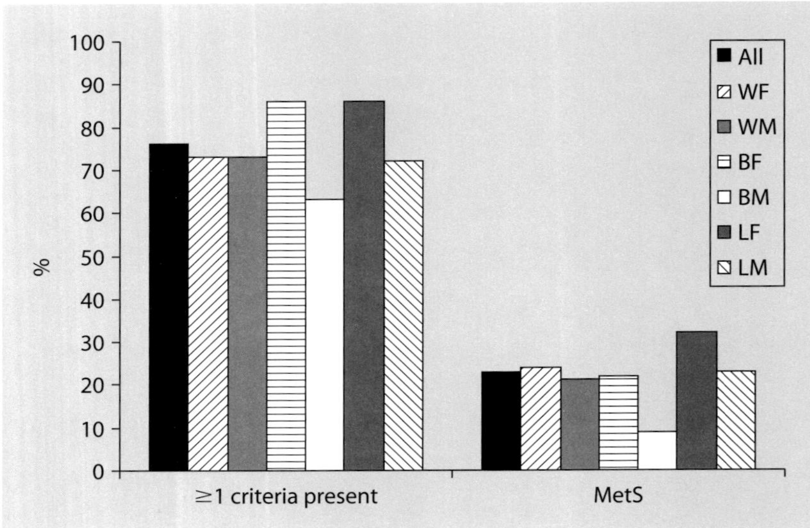

Fig. 2. Prevalence of MetS by race/gender (n = 1,028 patients with all MetS measures available). WF = White female, WM = white male, BF = black female, BM = black male, LF = Latina female, LM = Latino male, WC = waist circumference >102 cm for men or >88 cm for women, Trig = triglycerides ≥150 mg/dl, HDL cholesterol <40 mg/dl for men or <50 mg/dl for women, FBS = fasting blood sugar ≥110 mg/dl, HTN = hypertension diagnosis.

receiving medication for DM). However, the majority of patients with FBS ≥110 (76.0%, n = 187) were not receiving medications for DM, and 61.8% (n = 152) of this group did not have a recorded DM diagnosis during the index admission. Of the patients with a DM diagnosis, many were not receiving DM medication (44.2%, n = 84); for nearly half (45.7%, n = 37) in this subgroup FBS was ≥110 and in 21 FBS was >125. The majority of patients (71.6%, n = 748) without a diagnosis or medication for dyslipidemia did not have elevated triglycerides and did not meet the MetS criterion for elevated triglycerides. However, nearly half of patients with a recorded diagnosis of dyslipidemia (n = 105, 49.8%) were not receiving a statin, and 78.7% (n = 322) of those with triglycerides ≥150 did not have a diagnosis of dyslipidemia.

Discussion

Prevalence

The prevalence of MetS in this sample was significantly greater than in the general US population [19] but substantially lower than that reported in other studies of depressed patients. Rates as high as 57.9% have been found [2], but as noted above it is difficult to compare studies because prevalence can be affected by a number of variables, including the MetS criteria applied and the demographics of the sample. Since in clinical practice the emphasis is on identifying patients with any metabolic disturbance, not just those who have the full syndrome [28], the more important finding in the present study may be that at least one MetS criterion was present in a majority of patients (63.6–75.6%).

Treatment Variables Associated with MetS

A number of treatment variables were associated with increased risk for MetS, but, in contrast to previous reports, an association with atypical antipsychotics was not found. This result suggests that factors other than atypical antipsychotic exposure are important contributors to MetS in MDD, although this finding may not apply to other diagnostic groups. It is possible that prescribers at the study site selected antipsychotics with lower relative risks for metabolic side effects, perhaps especially in overweight patients or others considered at high risk for MetS. Consistent with this interpretation is that patients meeting the WC criterion were more likely to receive aripiprazole or ziprasidone, the atypical antipsychotics least associated with MetS [29], and less likely to be on drugs that block 5HTC2 (olanzapine, mirtazapine).

In contrast to the extensive literature about atypical antipsychotics and MetS, there are few published data about antidepressants and alterations in metabolic functions. (See the recent review by the investigators [13].) Most of these studies preceded the era of heightened awareness about the risk of MetS, and for those investigators weight gain was the only side effect addressed that was relevant to contemporary definitions of this syndrome. In the present study, both TCAs and venlafaxine were associated with increased risk on the triglyceride criterion, and the latter has been reported previously [30, 31]. Mirtazapine product labeling indicates that elevated triglycerides occur in ≤15% of patients [32]. Venlafaxine product labeling [30] notes the risk of elevated BP, but in the present study the only medication variables associated with the BP criterion were typical antipsychotics and receiving ≥2 antidepressants. Some SSRIs may also contribute to hypercholesterolemia (see, for example, Raeder et al. [33]), but the available data are limited and not conclusive.

A recent study of MetS in patients with bipolar disorder found statistically significant associations only for olanzapine/clozapine (p = < 0.001) and carbamazepine (negatively associated, p = 0.018) [34], suggesting that the 'mood stabilizers' (lithium, valproate, carbamazepine, lamotrigine, gabapentin) do not increase risk. However, many patients in this study who did not have MetS did meet the ATP III WC criterion. In addition, in the present study anticonvulsants as a class were associated with increased risk on the triglyceride and HDL measures, and weight gain is a well-known side effect of both lithium and valproate. Livingstone and Rampes [35] concluded that two-thirds of patients on lithium gain weight, and Perry et al. [36] reported a mean increase of 8.5 kg in patients treated for 6 months to 17 years.

There are little published data about lithium's effect on lipids; it may be associated with increased total cholesterol and triglycerides [37], but there have been no reports that suggest an effect on HDL. Lithium is not associated with increases in FBS or BP, although for patients who gain weight there may ultimately be secondary effects on other metabolic functions. Bowden's group recently reviewed the available data about weight gain associated with valproate and reported that there is an increase of 3–24 lb over a period of 3–12 months in up to 20% of patients [38, 39]. There are no reported associations with the cholesterol, triglyceride, FBS, or BP MetS criteria, but one study of prepubertal females with epilepsy found an increase in insulin resistance [40]. Reports about the effect of carbamazepine on weight are mixed [41–43] but do not suggest a potential for large increases in weight, and FBS and BP are not directly affected by carbamazepine. This drug is associated with increases in total cholesterol and HDL [38–40] and perhaps triglycerides as well [44]. Lamotrigine does not appear to be associated with weight gain, elevated FBS, or dyslipidemia [44–46]. The product labeling indicates that hypertension may occur [47], but there are no published reports of BP elevations. For gabapentin, there are no published studies which address its effects on cholesterol, triglycerides, or FBS. Product labeling states that FBS fluctuations and hypercholesterolemia are possible but adverse effects are rare [48]. There are no published reports of an association with elevated BP, but product labeling indicates that hypertension is a 'frequent' adverse effect (i.e. occurring in at least 1% of treated patients) [48]. Gabapentin's effect on weight appears to be variable; weight gain, which may be dose-dependent [49, 50], has only been studied in patients with epilepsy and headache [49–53].

Demographic Variables Associated with MetS

As demonstrated in the NHANES data, MetS findings in the general population vary by gender/race/ethnicity [4]. In the present study, the risk for MetS in Latino females was more than double that for other ethnic/gender categories, and the risk for females on the WC criterion was more than four times that for men. Also as expected, relatively older patients (in this case 40- to 59-year-olds) were at increased risk for the full syndrome and for four of the individual criteria: WC, triglycerides, FBS, and BP. Thus, the relative contributions of gender and race/ethnicity appear to be similar for both the general population [4] and this sample of depressed inpatients, although the overall prevalence of MetS and most of its individual criteria were greater in the latter.

Other Variables Associated with MetS

A number of mechanisms other than drug exposure have been proposed to explain the association between MetS and depression. Examples include chronic stress [6], excess cortisol [54–57], cytokine-mediated inflammation [10], a direct or indirect effect of insulin resistance [10], and products of adipose tissue such as leptin and tumor necrosis factor-α [54–57]. Severity and/or chronicity of depression may also be a factor. In one study, higher depression scores at baseline were associated with the later development of MetS [6], and in another study patients who remained depressed were more likely to develop MetS [2]. Several investigators have found associations between depression and the subsequent development of DM [2, 5, 58]. In the present study, illness severity, duration of illness, and length of treatment were not uniformly assessed, but several findings suggest that there was a high level of chronicity/severity in this sample. All subjects were inpatients at the time of enrollment, most (91.9%) had recurrent MDD as well as co-diagnoses on Axis I (70.2%) and/or Axis II (48.3%), and 36.5% had psychotic features. That most patients (77.2%) were treated with multiple psychotropics suggests a failure to respond fully to monotherapy, and treatment with ≥2 antidepressants, another potential indicator of relative treatment resistance, was associated with increased risk for MetS. In addition, a co-diagnosis of borderline personality disorder conferred increased risk for several MetS criteria, and data from STAR*D (Sequenced Treatment Alternatives to Relieve Depression) show higher rates of 'chronic depressive episodes' in black and Hispanic patients [56], subgroups with increased risks on several MetS measures in the present study.

Limitations

In interpreting the results of this study, it is important to note both the composition of the sample and the criteria used to define MetS. Although large and diverse, the sample did not represent all ages or ethnicities. All subjects were inpatients at the time of assessment, and a number of characteristics of the sample suggest that these patients may be more severely and/or chronically ill than those included in previous studies. Not all data were available on all patients, and reliable information was not available about smoking status, diet or exercise. The pharmacotherapy for these patients may not be representative of all clinical settings, and type and duration of medication exposure prior to the baseline assessment are not known. All patients were being treated for MDD, but diagnosis was not independently verified by the investigators. The variable 'diabetic medication', following the NHANES methodology [4], grouped all of the available pharmacotherapies for hyperglycemia. However, several recent studies have proposed that metformin, but not other oral hypoglycemics, may prevent the weight gain and insulin resistance associated with atypical antipsychotics [59–64]. Although the results from these trials have been mixed, it would have been preferable in the present study to control specifically for metformin rather than 'diabetic medication' generally in the regression analyses.

Conclusion

The study results indicate that atypical antipsychotics did not contribute to MetS in patients with depression. Furthermore, there is little to suggest that the majority of antidepressants and mood stabilizers play a major role in this syndrome. While no cause and effect relationships have been established, it is clear that many of the MDD patients in this clinical sample are at increased risk for MetS. Further research is needed to clarify the definition of metabolic syndrome and to refine tools for efficient and effective identification of at-risk patients in clinical settings. Future studies may inform drug development and guide treatment so that the metabolic status and vulnerabilities of the individual patient can be taken into account in the selection, dosing, and monitoring of pharmacotherapy.

References

1 Newcomer JW: Second generation (atypical) antipsychotics and metabolic effects: a comprehensive literature review. CNS Drugs 2005;19(suppl 1):1–93.

2 Heiskanen TH, Niskanen LK, Hintikka JJ, et al: Metabolic syndrome and depression: a cross-sectional analysis. J Clin Psychiatry 2006;67:1422–1427.

3 McEvoy JP, Meyer JM, Goff DC, et al: Prevalence of the metabolic syndrome in patients with schizophrenia: baseline results from the Clinical Antipsychotic Trials of Intervention Effectiveness (CATIE) schizophrenia trial and comparison with national estimates from NHANES III. Schizophr Res 2005;80:19–32.

4 Ford ES, Giles WH, Mokdad AH: Increasing prevalence of the metabolic syndrome among US adults. Diabetes Care 2004;27:2444–2449.

5 Kinder LS, Carnethon MR, Palaniappan LP, King AC, Fortmann SP: Depression and the metabolic syndrome in young adults: findings from the Third National Health and Nutrition Examination Survey. Psychosom Med 2004;66:316–322.

6 Raikkonen K, Matthews KA, Kuller LH: Depressive symptoms and stressful life events predict metabolic syndrome among middle-aged women. Diabetes Care 2007;30:872–877.

7 Goethe JW, Szarek BL, Woolley SB, Caley CF: Metabolic syndrome in psychiatric inpatients. Annual Meeting of the American Psychiatric Association, San Diego, 2007.

8 Everson-Rose SA, Meyer PM, Powell LH, et al: Depressive symptoms, insulin resistance, and risk of diabetes in women at midlife. Diabetes Care 2004;27:2856–2862.

9 Bryan CJ, Songer TJ, Brooks MM, et al: A comparison of baseline sociodemographic and clinical characteristics between major depressive disorder patients with and without diabetes: a STAR*D report. J Affect Disord 2008;108:113–120.

10 Koponen H, Jokelainen J, Keinanen-Kiukaanniemi S, Kumulsalo E, Vanhala M: Metabolic syndrome predisposes to depressive symptoms: a population-based 7-year follow-up study. J Clin Psychiatry 2008;69:178–182.

11 Skilton JR, Moulin P, Terra J-L, Bonnet F: Associations between anxiety, depression, and the metabolic syndrome. Biol Psychiatry 2007;62:1251–1257.

12 Grundy SM, Cleeman JI, Daniels SR, et al: Diagnosis and management of the metabolic syndrome: An American Heart Association/National Heart, and Blood Institute Scientific Statement. Circulation 2005;112:2735–2752.

13 Goethe JW, Szarek BL, Caley CF: Metabolic syndrome and depression: a review. Depression Mind Body 2008;3:138–149.

14 Third Report of the National Cholesterol Education Program (NCEP) Expert Panel on Detection, Evalulation, and Treatment of High Blood Cholesterol in Adults (Adult Treatment Panel III): Final Report. Circulation 2002;106:3143–3421.

15 Balkau B, Charles MA: Comment on the provisional report from the WHO consultation European Group for the Study of Insulin Resistance (EGIR). Diabet Med 1999;16:442–443.

16 Alberti KG, Zimmet P, Shaw J, IDF Epidemiology Task Force Consensus Group: The metabolic syndrome: a new worldwide definition. Lancet 2005;366:1059–1062.

17 Alberti KG, Zimmet PZ: Definition, diagnosis and classification of diabetes mellitus and its complications. 1. Diagnosis and classification of diabetes mellitus provisional report of a WHO consultation. Diabet Med 1998;15:539–553.
18 Einhorn D: ACE position statement on insulin resistance syndrome. Endocr Pract 2003;9:237–252.
19 Centers for Disease Control and Prevention (CDC): National Center for Health Statistics (NCHS). National Health and Nutrition Examination Survey Data. Hyattsville, MD: US Department of Health and Human Services, Centers for Disease Control and Prevention, 2003–2004, 222.edu.gov/nchs/nhames.htm.
20 Grundy SM, Benjamin IJ, Burke GL, et al: Diabetes and cardiovascular disease: a statement for healthcare professionals from the American Heart Association. Circulation 1999;100:1134–1146.
21 Kroeze WK, Hufeisen SJ, Popadak BA, Renock SM, Steinberg S, Ernsberger P, Jayathilake K, Meltzer HY, Roth BL: H1-histamine receptor affinity predicts short-term weight gain for typical and atypical antipsychotic drugs. Neuropsychopharmacology 2003;28:519–526.
22 Reynolds GP, Zhang AJ, Zhang XB: Association of antipsychotic drug-induced weight gain with a 5-HT2C receptor gene polymorphism. Lancet 2002;359:2086–2087.
23 Ellingrod VL, Perry PJ, Ringold JC, Lund BC, Bever-Stille K, Fleming F, Holman TL, Miller D: Weight gain with the –759 C/T polymorphism of the 5HT2C receptor and olanzapine. Am J Med Genet [B] 2005;134:76–78.
24 Wirshing DA, Wirshing WC, Kysar L, Berisford MA, Goldstein D, Pashdag J, Mintz J, Marder SR: Novel antipsychotics: comparison of weight gain liabilities. J Clin Psychiatry 1999;60:358–363.
25 Tecott LH, Sun LM, Akana SF, Strack AM, Lowenstein DH, Dallman MF, Julius D: Eating disorder and epilepsy in mice lacking 5-HT2C serotonin receptors. Nature 1995;374:542–546.
26 Newcomer JW: Antipsychotic medications: metabolic and cardiovascular risk. J Clin Psychiatry 2007;68(suppl 14):8–13.
27 American Diabetes Association, American Psychiatric Association, American Association of Clinical Endocrinologists, North American Association for the Study of Obesity: Consensus development conference on antipsychotic drugs and obesity and diabetes. J Clin Psychiatry 2004;65:267–272.
28 Grundy SM: Metabolic syndrome: a multiplex cardiovascular risk factor. J Clin Endocrinol Metab 2007;92:399–404.
29 Wirshing DA, Boyd JA, Meng LR, Ballon JS, Marder SR, Wirshing WC: The effects of novel antipsychotics on glucose and lipid levels. J Clin Psychiatry 2002;63:856–865.
30 Effexor Product Information. Wyeth Pharmaceuticals, Philadelphia, 2008.
31 Teitelbaum M: Severe hypertriglyceridemia secondary to venlafaxine and fluoxetine (letter to the editor). Psychosomatics 2001;42:440–441.
32 Organon: Remeron (mirtazapine) package insert. West Orange, Organon, 2001.
33 Raeder MB, Bjelland I, Vollset SE, Steen VM: Obesity, dyslipidemia, and diabetes with selective serotonin reuptake inhibitors: the Hordaland Health Study. J Clin Psychiatry 2006;67:1974–1982.
34 Cardenas J, Frye MA, Marusak SL, et al Modal subcomponents of metabolic syndrome in patients with bipolar disorder. J Affect Disord. 2008;106:91–97.
35 Livingstone C, Rampes H: Lithium: a review of its metabolic adverse effects. J Psychopharmacol 2006;20:347–355.
36 Anon: Mood stabilizers; in Perry PJ, Alexander B, Liskow BI, DeVane CL (eds): Psychotropic Drug Handbook. Philadelphia, Lippincott Williams & Wilkins, 2007, pp 226–295.
37 Fankhauser M, Kreuger R, Finley P: Triglyceride and cholesterol concentrations in serum during chronic lithium therapy: a retrospective comparison of baseline and follow-up laboratory values. Lithium 1991;2:77–81.
38 Bowden CL: Valproate. Bipolar Disorders 2003;5:189–202.
39 Bowden CL, Singh V: Valproate in bipolar disorder: 2000 onwards. Acta Psychiatr Scand 2005;111(suppl 426):13–20.
40 Verrotti A, Basciani F, De Simone M, Trotta D, Morgese G, Chiarelli F: Insulin resistance in epileptic girls who gain weight after therapy with valproic acid. J Child Neurol 2002;17:265–268.
41 Post RM, Ketter TA, Uhde T, Ballenger JC: Thirty years of clinical experience with carbamazepine in the treatment of bipolar illness: principles and practice. CNS Drugs 2007;21:47–71.
42 Weisler RH, Hirschfeld, Cutler AJ, Gazda T, Ketter TA, Keck PE, Swann A, Kalali A, et al: Extended-release carbamazepine capsules as monotherapy in bipolar disorder. Pooled results from two randomized, double-blind, placebo-controlled trials. CNS Drugs 2006;20:219–231.
43 Joffe RT, Post RM, Uhde TW: Effect of carbamazepine on body weight in affectively ill patients. J Clin Psychiatry 1986;47:313–314.
44 Brown DW, Ketter TA, Crumlish J, Post RM: Carbamazepine-induced increases in total serum cholesterol: clinical and theoretical implications. J Clin Psychopharmacol 1992;12:431–437.

45 Bowden CL, Calabrese JR, Ketter TA, Sachs GS, White RL, Thompson TR: Impact of lamotrigine and lithium on weight in obese and nonobese patients with bipolar I disorder. Am J Psychiatry 2006;163:1199–1201.
46 Brown EB, McElroy SL, Keck PE, Deldar A, Adams DH, Tohen M, et al: A 7-week, randomized, double-blind trial of olanzapine/fluoxetine combination versus lamotrigine in the treatment of bipolar I depression. J Clin Psychiatry 2006;67:1025–1033.
47 Lamictal Product Information. Research Triangle Park, Glaxo Smith Kline, 2007.
48 Neurontin Product Information. New York, Pfizer Pharmaceuticals, 2005.
49 Morris GL: Gabapentin. Epilepsia 1999;40(suppl 5):S63–S70.
50 DeToledo JC, Toledo C, DeCerce J, Ramsay RE: Changes in body weight with chronic, high-dose gabapentin therapy. Ther Drug Monit 1997;19:394–396.
51 Ben-Menachem E: Weight issues for people with epilepsy: a review. Epilepsia 2007;48(suppl 9):42–45.
52 Maggioni F, Ruffatti S, Dainese F, Mainardi F, Zanchin G: Weight variations in the prophylactic therapy of primary headaches: 6-month follow-up. J Headache Pain 2005;6:322–324.
53 Jallon P, Picard F: Bodyweight gain and anticonvulsants: a comparative review. Drug Saf 2001;24:969–978.
54 Pasco JA, Jacka FN, Williams LJ, et al: Leptin in depressed women: cross sectional and longitudinal data from an epidemiologic study. J Affect Disord 2008;107:221–225.
55 Vestri HS, Maianu L, Moellering DR, Garvey WT: Atypical antipsychotic drugs directly impair insulin action in adipocytes: effects on glucose transport, lipogenesis, and antilipolysis (see comment). Neuropsychopharmacology 2007;32:765–772.
56 Gilmer WS, Trivedi MH, Rush AJ, Wisniewski SR, Luther J, Howland RH, Yohanna D, Khan A, Alpert J: Factors associated with chronic depressive episodes: a preliminary report from the STAR-D project. Acta Psychiatr Scand 2005;112:425–433.
57 Brown ES, Varghese FP, McEwen BS: Association of depression with medical illness: does cortisol play a role? Biol Psychiatry 2004;55:1–9.
58 Carnethon MR, Biggs ML, Barzilay JI, et al: Longitudinal association between depressive symptoms and incident type 2 diabetes mellitus in older adults: the cardiovascular health study. Arch Intern Med 2007;167:802–807.
59 Baptista T, Martinez J, Lacruz AN, et al: Metformin for prevention of weight gain and insulin resistance with olanzapine: a double-blind placebo-controlled trial. Can J Psychiatry 2006;51:192–196.
60 Wu R-R, Zhao J-P, Jin H, Shao P, Fang M-S, Guo X-F, et al: Lifestyle intervention and metformin for treatment of antipsychotic-induced weight gain: a randomized controlled trial. JAMA 2008;299:185–193.
61 Baptista T, Sandia I, Lacruz A, et al: Insulin counter-regulatory factors, fibrinogen and C-reactive protein during olanzapine administration: effects of the antidiabetic metformin. Int Clin Psychopharmacol 2007;22:69–76.
62 Baptista T, Rangel N, Fernandez V, et al: Metformin as an adjunctive treatment to control body weight and metabolic dysfunction during olanzapine administration: a multicentric, double-blind, placebo-controlled trial. Schizophr Res 2007;93:99–108.
63 Klein DJ, Cottingham EM, Sorter M, Barton BA, Morrison JA: A randomized, double-blind, placebo-controlled trial of metformin treatment of weight gain associated with initiation of atypical antipsychotic therapy in children and adolescents. Am J Psychiatry 2006;163:2072–2079.
64 Gaede P, Lund-Andersen H, Parving H-H, Pedersen O: Effect of a multifactorial intervention on mortality in type 2 diabetes. N Engl J Med 2008;358:580–591.

John W. Goethe, MD
Institute of Living
200 Retreat Avenue
Hartford, CT 06106 (USA)
Tel. +1 (860) 545 7118, Fax +1 (860) 545 7066, E-Mail jgoethe@harthosp.org

Thakore J, Leonard BE (eds): Metabolic Effects of Psychotropic Drugs.
Mod Trends Pharmacopsychiatry. Basel, Karger, 2009, vol 26, pp 105–115

Hyperprolactinaemia Associated with Antipsychotic Medications

Peter Fitzgerald · Timothy G. Dinan

Department of Psychiatry and Alimentary Pharmabiotic Centre, University College, Cork, Ireland

Abstract

Hyperprolactinaemia is now recognised as one of the most common adverse effects of antipsychotic medications. It is a potentially serious adverse outcome associated with significant morbidity, but can be clinically silent for many years. This chapter firstly outlines the predominant regulatory mechanism involved in prolactin secretion, that of dopaminergic inhibition of the pituitary lactotrope, and thereafter discusses the pathophysiology of antipsychotic-induced hyperprolactinaemia. All antipsychotic medications can affect prolactin levels via binding to dopamine receptors on the lactotrope cell membrane, with those which have potent D2 receptor antagonism and poorest blood-brain permeability having the greatest and most sustained effect. Those medications which easily cross the blood-brain barrier and exhibit fast dissociation from the dopamine receptor once bound have the least impact on serum prolactin concentrations. Given the potential serious adverse effects of hyperprolactinaemia for patients in both the short-term (sexual dysfunction, amenorrhoea, galactorrhoea) and long-term (osteopenia and osteoporosis, increased risk of hip fracture, possibly increased risk of certain cancers and tumours), the clinician should be alert to its occurrence in those prescribed antipsychotic medications, particularly of the typical and prolactin-elevating atypical variety.

In recent years, there has been a growing awareness of the higher risk of a range of physical illnesses in patients with long-term mental illness [1–3] and consideration of the risk of physical disease complications must now be a prominent factor when selecting treatments for mental illness [4].

Hyperprolactinaemia is now recognised as one of the most common adverse effects of antipsychotic medications. It is a potentially serious adverse outcome, associated with significant morbidity such as hypogonadism leading to osteoporosis and increased risk of hip fracture [5], and a growing body of evidence has linked elevations in prolactin to a possible increased risk of certain cancers (breast most notably, but also prostate) and pituitary tumours [6–10]. However, until relatively recently, this common endocrine problem has been under-reported and under-researched within the psychiatric scientific community. It may be clinically silent for many years, or its commonest symptoms of sexual dysfunction may be undisclosed by the patient [11] or indeed erroneously ascribed to the underlying disease process rather than as an adverse effect of medication. Concerns regarding the possible impact of persistent hyperprolactinaemia are only recently coming into focus as the widespread use of atypical antipsychotics as 1st line agents has shifted attention away from the main problems of their forerunners (those of extra-pyramidal side effects and tardive dyskinesia) to newer concerns regarding metabolic and endocrine abnormalities, including hyperprolactinaemia.

Although it had been recognised since the early 1960s that typical antipsychotic medications could cause amenorrhoea and galactorrhoea, it was not until the mid-1970s, with the advent of radio-immune assays which allowed for the accurate measurement of prolactin (PRL), that raised levels were consistently demonstrated in the majority of medication-treated patients with schizophrenia [12, 13]. All typical antipsychotic agents are associated with raised PRL levels by virtue of their antagonism of the dopamine receptor (see below), and of the newer, atypical medications, there is great disparity in terms of their effect on PRL, with some having a minor, transient impact on levels while others display a profoundly elevating effect greater than any of the traditional agents.

The focus of this chapter is firstly to provide an outline of the dopaminergic regulation of PRL synthesis and secretion, which will provide a framework for understanding the mechanism of action of antipsychotics in causing hyperprolactinaemia, and furthermore to discuss the possible reasons why some atypical medications are 'prolactin-sparing' while others are strongly 'prolactin-elevating.'

Prolactin

PRL is a polypeptide hormone that is predominantly synthesized and secreted from lactotrope cells of the anterior pituitary gland. It was discovered by Riddle et al. [14] in 1933 who demonstrated its ability to elicit lactation in mammals, and though it has since been found to have numerous other diverse physiological functions (over 300 different biological actions in vertebrates), it remains best known, and continues to take its name from, this function.

The predominant control of PRL synthesis and secretion is via dopaminergic inhibitory input to the lactotrope cells from the hypothalamus. This tonic upstream inhibition conveys a unique characteristic to PRL secretion compared to the other pituitary hormones, whose secretory tone is largely determined by stimulatory agents. This discrepancy stems from prolactin's lack of a single target organ to provide a classical negative feedback loop (in contrast to, for example, adrenocorticotropin hormone). Also, lactotropes have much higher basal secretory activity compared to other endocrine cells, and are thus more responsive to inhibition than stimulation.

Prolactin Structure

Prolactin belongs to a large family of proteins known as group I of the helix bundle protein hormones [15], other members of which include growth hormone, placental lactogen and a multitude of prolactin-related proteins. All genes encoding this group share a certain degree of homology (e.g. 40% homology between PRL and GH genes) due to their evolution from a single common ancestral gene approximately 400 million years ago [16]. Such homogeneity leads to a certain degree of functional overlap between group members, such as the capability of human GH to bind to the PRL receptor and thus to mimic some of PRL's actions. PRL, however, has a much more diverse spectrum of action compared to GH, being involved in a broad array of functions extending from reproduction and lactation to roles in metabolism, behaviour, immunoregulation and osmoregulation [17].

Humans possess a single PRL gene on chromosome 6 [18], the expression of which primarily occurs in the pituitary gland, although multiple extra-pituitary sites also express the gene where different (tissue-specific) regulatory mechanisms are in place [19]. The structure of the PRL molecule follows a single chain of amino acids with 3 intramolecular disulfide bonds between 6 cysteine residues. Although the major form of PRL found in the pituitary consists of 199 amino acids with a molecular mass of approximately 23 kDa, multiple variants of it have been characterised in humans through processes such as alternative splicing, proteolytic cleavage, and other post-translational modifications [20].

Location of Synthesis and Secretion

The predominant site of synthesis and secretion of PRL is the anterior pituitary gland, where specialized pituicytes known as lactotropes synthesize and release the hormone. Dependent on their location within the gland, lactotropes display marked functional heterogeneity in their response to secretagogues: those located in the outer zone are more responsive to thyrotropinreleasing hormone (TRH), a potent hypothalamic prolactin releasing factor, while those in the inner zone are more response to the inhibitory action of dopamine [21,22].

Though the anterior pituitary lies outside of the blood-brain barrier, PRL has been observed in several brain structures, most notably the hypothalamus, cerebral cortex, limbic system, and brain stem [23–26]. The source of this brain prolactin remains predominantly pituitary derived, gaining access to the CNS via the choroid plexi, although the hypothalamus is also capable of synthesizing an identical variant of the hormone [24].

Additional peripheral sites of synthesis of the hormone include the placenta, decidua and myometrium of the non-pregnant uterus, the epithelial cells of the lactating mammary gland and in lymphocytes [20] where its synthesis and secretion are under tissue-specific regulatory factors outside of the scope of this discussion.

Prolactin Receptors and Signalling

The prolactin receptor is a transmembrane protein which belongs to class 1 of the cytokine receptor superfamily [27]. The gene encoding this receptor is found on chromosome 5 in humans, and alternative splicing produces 3 major PRL-R isoforms based on amino acid sequence, the short, intermediate and long forms, with the latter being the main isoform through which PRL transmits its signals. Each protein consists of an identical extracellular domain, a short transmembrane domain and a variable intracellular domain that mediates signalling.

The receptors are devoid of any intrinsic tyrosine kinase activity but once activated can be phosphorylated by cytoplasmic proteins. Binding of PRL to its receptor activates several signalling pathways, the main one being the Janus-kinase-Signal transducer and activator of transcription (Jak-Stat) pathway, while others include the MAPK and the phosphoinositide 3 kinase pathway.

It is generally accepted that activation of the receptor involves ligand-induced sequential receptor dimerization. Initially, PRL binds to a single transmembrane receptor, forming an inactive hormone-receptor complex which then binds a second receptor leading to receptor dimerization and activation of a cascade of secondary messenger systems [28] (fig. 1).

Within the hypothalamus, both long and short receptor isoforms are expressed, and are particularly prominent within the arcuate and periventricular nuclei [29]. These regions play an integral part in orchestrating the inhibitory dopaminergic tone which the hypothalamus provides to the lactotrope, and the expression of PRL receptors in these nuclei allows PRL to participate in a feedback mechanism which helps to regulate its own secretion (termed 'short-loop feedback regulation'; fig. 2).

Dopamine's Regulation of Prolactin

A large corpus of research has upheld dopamine's predominant role in the regulation of prolactin synthesis and secretion. The tuberoinfundibular dopaminergic (TIDA) neuronal population, the cell bodies of which reside in the arcuate nucleus of the hypothalamus, is the most important in regulating PRL release in humans [30]. Neurons from TIDA population project to the external zone of the medial eminence, where they release DA into the perivascular spaces surrounding the capillary loops. From here, dopamine travels along the long portal veins to the anterior lobe of the pituitary (fig. 2), where it has a direct effect on lactotropes by binding to the dopamine type 2 receptor expressed on their cell membranes [31]. Activation of this receptor results in the suppression of both PRL gene expression and inhibition of hormone exocytosis [32–34].

In addition to its direct effect on prolactin at the level of the pituitary, there is some evidence for an effect of central dopaminergic tone on PRL secretion also, such as

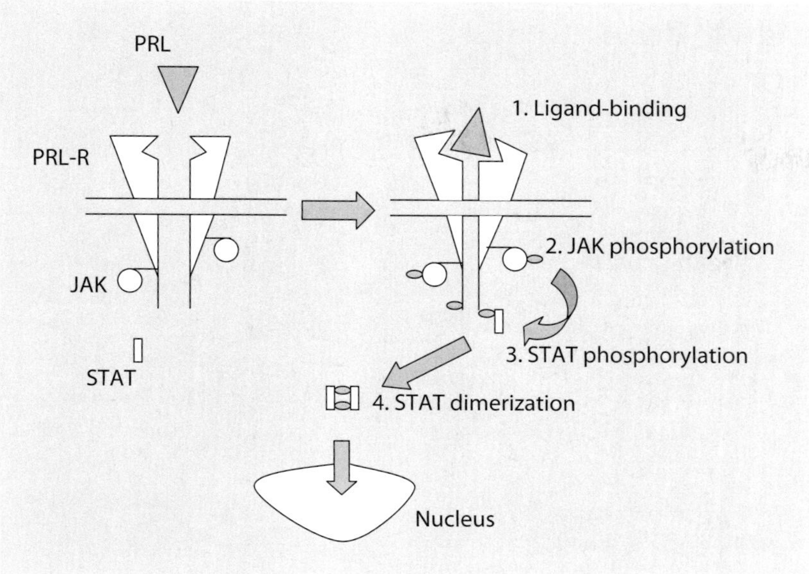

Fig. 1. The principle signalling pathway of prolactin. Step 1: PRL molecule binds to receptor, initiating and so on receptor dimerization. Step 2: Receptor activation leads to tyrosine kinase (JAK) phosphorylation, which is subsequently responsible for the phosphorylation of a signal transducer and activator of transcription (STAT) protein when it docks to the activated receptor (step 3). The activated STAT molecule then dissociates from the receptor complex and forms a dimer with another phosphorylated STAT protein (step 4), which then translocates to the nucleus to initiate target gene transcription (e.g. increase tyrosine hydroxylase induction in TIDA neurons).

the finding from rodent studies of a dopamine type 1 receptor-mediated decrease in TIDA activity [35, 36], although the physiological significance of such findings are as of yet uncertain and of less importance than the principle peripheral effect of dopamine on the lactotrope.

In the absence of target gland hormones to provide feedback control over the lactotropes, PRL is capable of regulating its own release by modulating the hypothalamic dopaminergic neurons of the arcuate nucleus via a short loop negative feedback mechanism (fig. 2). The hypothalamus is one of the highest density regions within the brain for expression of the PRL-R, and it has been demonstrated that PRL-R colocalizes with neurons expressing tyrosine hydroxylase, the rate-limiting enzyme in dopamine synthesis [37]. Both enzyme activation [38] and induction [39] have been observed as a direct result of PRL's action on these neurons, and this effect has been shown to be exclusively dependent on the STAT5b protein-mediated signal transduction component of the JAK-STAT pathway [40]. Furthermore, PRL's stimulatory effect on dopaminergic neurons seems to be quite specific to the hypothalamus as indicated by the finding that hyperprolactinaemia augments TH mRNA levels in the arcuate nucleus but not the substantia nigra [39].

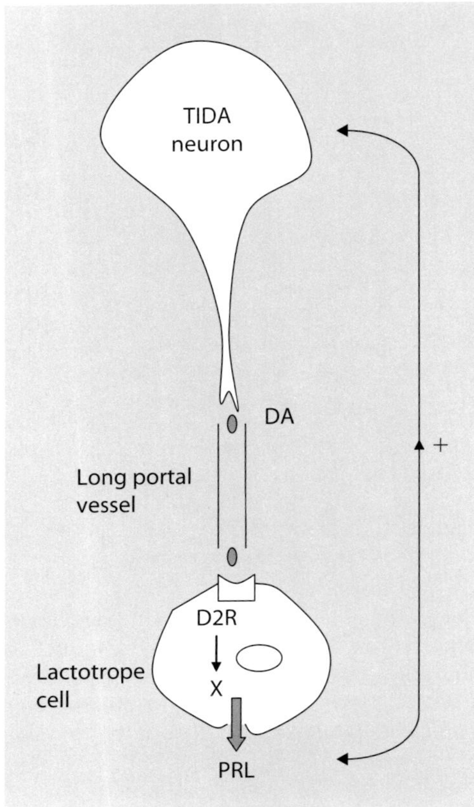

Fig. 2. The short-loop feedback mechanism of prolactin regulation. PRL released from pituitary lactotropes feeds back to the tuberoinfundibular dopaminergic neuronal population of the hypothalamus, where binding to its cell surface receptor initiates a signalling cascade which ultimately increases dopamine synthesis within the neuron. Dopamine travels back to the anterior pituitary via long portal veins, where it binds to D2 receptors on the lactotrope and inhibits synthesis and secretion of PRL.

It is thought that the predominant source of PRL which participates in short-loop feedback is pituitary derived, reaching the arcuate nuclei by either retrograde blood flow from the pituitary or from the CSF which it enters via the choroid plexus [41, 42].

Antipsychotic-Induced Hyperprolactinaemia

Typical Antipsychotics

Typical antipsychotic medications such as haloperidol or chlorpromazine are a class of older medications developed in the 1950s whose efficacy as antipsychotic agents is defined by their potency in blocking the dopamine type 2 receptors in the brain.

They were first shown to stimulate PRL release by Clemens and colleagues in 1974 [12] and it is now widely recognised that all typical antipsychotics can be associated with sustained elevations in PRL. The principle method of action for this is by diminishing the influence of dopamine on the lactotrope via D2 receptor blockade on the cell membrane. Furthermore, due to the tight binding of these typical drugs to the dopamine receptor, they dissociate slowly from it and thus result in a more prolonged receptor blockade which can lead to a cumulative effect on PRL levels from one dose to the next [43].

Prevalence rates of hyperprolactinaemia in patients prescribed typical antipsychotics are high, with estimations ranging from 33% to over 80% [44, 45]. The large discrepancy between studies is most probably best explained by differing dosages, with lower doses being associated with less of a propensity for elevated PRL due to less receptor occupancy. In relation to depot formulations, recent naturalistic studies have reported hyperprolactinaemia in approximately 35% of patients [44, 46].

Atypical Antipsychotics

The 'atypical' antipsychotic medications encompass a heterogeneous group of compounds which vary significantly in terms of their D2 receptor blocking potency, with some having weak antagonist properties for the receptor (e.g. clozapine) while others display potent D2 antagonism (e.g. risperidone, amisulpride). Therefore, classification of antipsychotic drugs as typical or atypical has little relevance to the relative propensity of these agents to cause hyperprolactinaemia.

Of the newer second-generation medications, most are not implicated in significant sustained increases of PRL and are thus known as 'prolactin-sparing' (e.g. clozapine, quetiapine, olanzapine and aripiprazole fall into this class of antipsychotic). Two further atypicals, however (risperidone and amisulpride), have a significant PRL elevating property more like those of the typical variety [47], demonstrating that D2 receptor potency of the compound is the most cogent factor when predicting the compound's effect on PRL levels.

Another relevant consideration is the relative brain permeability of the medication, with those with poor permeability across the blood-brain barrier being more likely to cause hyperprolactinaemia. In rodents, atypical antipsychotics with a propensity for prolactin elevation have been shown to display much greater pituitary versus central D2 receptor occupancy than those which are prolactin-sparing [48], and compounds which had the highest peripheral-to-central potency displayed the greatest PRL elevation. Relative difficulty getting across the blood-brain barrier hence seems to be of importance with respect to an atypicals effect on prolactin release since higher doses will be required to effect a given level of central dopamine occupancy, a result of which is a higher number of peripheral pituitary D2 receptors also being blocked.

It should be borne in mind that all antipsychotics result in at least a transient increase in prolactin levels in humans – even those classified as prolactin-sparing demonstrate a non-sustained elevation, and this can result in an abnormal serum prolactin measurement depending on the timing of the blood test subsequent to that of the last dose administered. The difference between prolactin-sparing and prolactin-elevating compounds is not qualitative but rather in the sustained nature of the increase in the latter group [49]. The transient increase in PRL found with medications such as clozapine and quetiapine results from the fast dissociation of the compound from the D2 receptor over a matter of hours following dose administration. Studies demonstrate a steep fall in receptor occupancy for these agents from approximately 60% within 2 h of administration of a mid-range dose to less than 30% at 24 h [50–52] thus negating any possible cumulative effect on PRL of subsequent doses.

Prevalence rates of hyperprolactinaemia in patients prescribed atypical antipsychotic agents vary significantly according to the individual drug and dependent on its properties as outlined above. Most studies which report prolactin levels do so not as a primary outcome measure but rather as part of the set of laboratory parameters assessed in research aimed at efficacy measurement, and as such provide point-prevalence figures only which do not take into account the transient nature of PRL elevation incurred after some antipsychotic administration or assess persistence. Nevertheless, amisulpride seems to be associated with the highest risk of hyperprolactinaemia with point-prevalence rates of 80–100% reported in the literature [44, 53, 54]. Risperidone is also associated with hyperprolactinaemia in the majority who take it, with rates ranging from 70 to 100% of cases consistently reported [55–57]. Of atypicals which are known to be 'prolactin-sparing' in nature, rates range from less than 5 to approximately 30%, but the possibility of measuring prolactin during a transient peak soon after dose administration was not accounted for in any studies [53].

Conclusions

By virtue of dopamine's direct peripheral effect on the D2 receptor of cells within the anterior pituitary gland, the basally high secretory tone of the lactotrope is curtailed and prolactin levels are kept to homeostatic levels. The predominant regulator of the dopaminergic neurons involved in this pathway is itself prolactin, which feeds back to the hypothalamus and stimulates increased dopamine production within the tuberoinfundibular neuronal population, thus completing a feedback mechanism in controlling its own synthesis and secretion.

All antipsychotic medications can affect prolactin levels via binding to dopamine receptors on the lactotrope cell membrane, with those which have potent D2 receptor antagonism and poorest blood-brain permeability having the greatest and most sustained effect. Those medications which easily cross the blood-brain barrier and exhibit fast dissociation from the dopamine receptor once bound have the least impact on serum prolactin concentrations.

Given the potential serious adverse effects of hyperprolactinaemia for patients in both the short-term (sexual dysfunction, amenorrhoea, galactorrhoea) and long-term (osteopenia and osteoporosis, increased risk of hip fracture, possibly increased risk of certain cancers and tumours), the clinician should be alert to its occurrence in those prescribed antipsychotic medications, particularly of the typical and prolactin-elevating atypical variety.

Future research is needed in this area through large prospective cohort studies to clarify more accurately the risk factors, prevalence and consequences of hyperprolactinaemia within antipsychotic-treated patients.

References

1 Brown S, Inskip H, Barraclough B: Causes of the excess mortality of schizophrenia. Br J Psychiatry 2000;177:212–217.

2 Dalton SO, Mellemkjaer L, Thomassen L, Mortensen PB, Johansen C: Risk for cancer in a cohort of patients hospitalized for schizophrenia in Denmark, 1969–1993. Schizophr Res 2005;75:315–324.

3 Osborn DJP, Levy G, Nazareth I, Peterson I, Islam A, King MB: Relative risk of cardiovascular and cancer mortality in people with severe mental illness from the United Kingdom's General Practice Research Database. Arch Gen Psychiatry 2007; 64:242–249.

4 Dinan TG, Thakore J, Citrome L, Gough SCL, Haddad P, Holt RIG, O'Donovan MC, Paton C, Peveler R, Yoemans D, Young I, Pendlebury J: Metabolic and lifestyle issues and severe mental illness: new connections to well-being? J Psychopharmacol 2005;19(suppl):118–122.

5 Howard L, Kirkwood G, Lesse M: Risk of hip fracture in patients with a history of schizophrenia. Br J Psychiatry 2007;190:129–134.

6 Tworoger SS, Eliassen AH, Rosner B, Sluss P, Hankinson SE: Plasma prolactin concentrations and risk of postmenopausal breast cancer. Cancer Res 2004;64:6814–6819.

7 Wang PS, Walker AM, Tsuang MT: Dopamine antagonists and the development of breast cancer. Arch Gen Psychiatry 2002;59:1147–1154.

8 Tworoger SS, Eliassen H, Sluss P, Hankinson S: A prospective study of plasma prolactin concentrations and risk of premenopausal and postmenopausal breast cancer. J Clin Oncol 2007;25: 1482–1488.

9 Szarfman A, Tonning JM, Levine JG, Doraiswamy PM: Atypical antipsychotics and pituitary tumours: a pharmacovigilance study. Pharmacotherapy 2006; 26:748–758.

10 Harvey PW, Everett DJ, Springall CJ: Adverse effects of prolactin in rodents and humans: breast and prostate cancer. J Psychopharmacol 2008; 22(suppl): 20–27.

11 Wesselmann U, Windgassen K: Galactorrhea: subjective response by schizophrenic patients. Acta Psychiatr Scand 1995;91:152–155.

12 Clemens, JA, Smalstig EB, Sawyer BD: Antipsychotic drugs stimulate prolactin release. Psychopharmacology 1974;40:123–127.

13 Meltzer HY, Sachar EJ, Frantz AG: Serum Prolactin Levels in Newly Admitted Psychiatric Patients: Neuropsychopharmacology of Monoamines and Their Regulatory Enzymes. New York, Raven Press, 1974.

14 Riddle O, Bates RW, Dykshorn SW: The preparation, identification and assay of prolactin: a hormone of the anterior pituitary. Am J Physiol 1933; 105:191–216.

15 Horseman ND and Yu-Lee LY: Transcriptional regulation by the helix bundle peptide hormones: growth hormone, prolactin, and hematopoietic cytokines. Endocr Rev 1994;15:627–649.

16 Cooke NE, Corr D, Shine J, Baxter JD, Martial JA: Human prolactin cDNA structural analysis and evolutionary comparisons. J Biol Chem 1981;256: 4007–4016.

17 Goffin V, Binart N, Touraine P, Kelly PA: Prolactin: the new biology of an old hormone. Annu Rev Physiol 2002;64:47–67.

18 Owerbach D, Rutter WJ, Cooke NE, Martial JA, Shows TB: The prolactin gene is located on chromosome 6 in humans. Science 1981;212:815–816.

19 Ben Jonathan N, Mershon JL, Allen DL, Steinmetz RW: Extrapituitary prolactin: distribution, regulation, functions, and clinical aspects. Endocr Rev 1996;17:639–669.

20 Freeman ME, Kanyicska B, Lerant A, Nagy G: Prolactin: structure, function, and regulation of secretion. Physiol Rev 2000:80:1523–1631.

21 Boockfor FR, Frawley LS: Functional variations among prolactin cells from different pituitary regions. Endocrinology 1987;120:874–879.

22 Arita J, Kojima Y, Kimura F: Identification by the sequential cell immunoblot assay of a subpopulation of rat dopamine-unresponsive lactotrophs. Endocrinology 1991;128:1887–1894.

23 Fuxe K, Hokfelt T, Eneroth P, Gustafsson JA, Skett P: Prolactin-like immunoreactivity: localization in nerve terminals of rat hypothalamus. Science 1977; 196:899–900.

24 DeVito WJ: Distribution of immunoreactive prolactin in the male and female rat brain: effects of hypophysectomy and intraventricular administration of colchicines. Neuroendocrinology 1988;47:284–289.

25 Seroogy K, Tsuruo Y, Hokfelt T, Walsh J, Fahrenkrug J, Emson PC, Goldstein M: Further analysis of presence of peptides in dopamine neurons: cholecystokinin, peptide histidine-isoleucine/vasoactive intestinal peptide and substance P in rat supramamillary region and mesencephalon. Exp Brain Res 1988;72:523–534.

26 Harlan RE, Shivers BD, Fox SR, Kaplove KA, Schachter BS, Pfaff SW: Distribution and partial characterization of immunoreactive prolactin in the rat brain. Neuroendocrinology 1989;49:7–22.

27 Bazan JF: Structural design and molecular evolution of a cytokine receptor superfamily. Proc Natl Acad Sci USA 1990;87:6934–6938.

28 Bole-Feysot C, Goffin V, Edery M, Binart N, Kelly PA: Prolactin (PRL) and its receptor: actions, signal transduction pathways and phenotypes observed in PRL receptor knockout mice. Endocr Rev 1998;19:225–268.

29 Pi XJ, Grattan DR: Differential expression of the two forms of prolactin receptor mRNA within microdissected hypothalamic nuclei of the rat. Brain Res Mol Brain Res 1998;59:1–12.

30 Ben-Jonathan N, Hnasko R: Dopamine as a prolactin (PRL) inhibitor. Endocr Rev 2001;22:724–763.

31 Caron MC, Beaulieu M, Raymond V, Gange B, Drouin J, Lefkowitz J, Labrie F: Dopaminergic receptors in the anterior pituitary gland. J Biol Chem 1978;253:2244.

32 Enjalbert A, Bockaert J: Pharmacological characterization of D2 dopamine receptors negatively coupled with adenylate cyclase in the rat anterior pituitary. Mol Pharmacol 1983;23:576–584.

33 Enjalbert A, Guillon G, Mouillac B, Audinot V, Rasolonjanahary R, Kordon C, Bockaert J: Dual mechanisms of inhibition by dopamine of basal and thyrotropin-releasing hormone-stimulated inositol phosphate production in anterior pituitary cells: evidence for an inhibition not mediated by voltage-dependent calcium channels. J Biol Chem 1990;265:18816–18822.

34 Lledo PM, Israel JM, Vincent JD: Chronic stimulation of D2 dopamine receptors specifically inhibits calcium but not potassium currents in rat lactotrophs. Brain Res 1991;558:231–238.

35 Berry SA, Gudelsky GA: D1 receptors function to inhibit the activation of tuberoinfundibular dopamine neurons. J Pharmacol Exp Ther 1990;254:677–682.

36 Durham RA, Eaton MJ, Moore KE, Lookingland KJ: Effects of selective activation of dopamine D2 and D3 receptors on prolactin secretion and the activity of tuberoinfundibular dopamine neurons. Eur J Pharmacol 1997;335:37–42.

37 Arbogast LA, Voogt JL: Prolactin (PRL) receptors are colocalized in dopaminergic neurons in fetal hypothalamic cell cultures: effect of PRL on tyrosine hydroxylase activity. Endocrinology 1997;138:3016–3023.

38 Pasqualini C, Bojda F, Gaudoux F, Guibert B, Leviel V, Teissier E, Rips R, Kerdelhue B: Changes in tuberoinfundibular dopaminergic neuron activity during the rat estrous cycle in relation to the prolactin surge: alteration by a mammary carcinogen. Neuroendocrinology 1988;48:320–327.

39 Arbogast LA, Voogt JL: Hyperprolactinaemia increases and hypoprolactinaemia decreases tyrosine hydroxylase messenger ribonucleic acid levels in the arcuate nuclei, but not the substantia nigra or zona incerta. Endocrinology 1991;128:997–1005.

40 Ma FY, Anderson GM, Gunn TD, Goffin V, Grattan DR, Bunn SJ: Prolactin specifically activates signal transducer and activator of transcription 5b in neuroendocrine dopaminergic neurons. Endocrinology 2005;146:5112–5119.

41 Oliver C, Mical RS, Porter JC: Hypothalamic-pituitary vasculature: evidence for retrograde blood flow in the pituitary stalk. Endocrinology 1977; 101:598–604.

42 Mangurian LP, Walsh RJ, Posner BI: Prolactin enhancement of its own uptake at the choroid plexus. Endocrinology 1992;131:698–702.

43 Seeman P: Atypical antipsychotics: mechanisms of action. Can J Psych 2002;47:27–38.

44 Bushe C, Shaw M: Prevalence of hyperprolactinaemia in a naturalistic cohort of schizophrenia and bipolar outpatients during treatment with typical and atypical antipsychotics. J Psychopharmacol 2008; 21:768–773.

45 Jakovljevic M, Pivac N, Mihaljevic-Peles A, Mustapic M, Relja M, Ljubicic D, Marcinko D, Muck-Seler D: The effects of olanzapine and fluphenazine on plasma cortisol, prolactin and muscle rigidity in schizophrenic patients: a double blind study. Prog Neuropsychopharmacol Biol Psychiatry 2007;31: 399–402.

46 Crockett A, Goldstein M, Bushe C: How has NICE guidelines affected prescribing in depot clinic schizophrenia outpatients? The Dewsbury Experience. British Association of Psychopharmacology 2005 Summer Meeting 24–27 July, Harrogate, 2005.

47 Stanniland C, Taylor D: Tolerability of atypical antipsychotics. Drug Saf 2000;22:195–214.

48 Kapur S, Langlois X, Vinken P, Megens AAHP, De Coster R, Andrews JS: The differential effects of atypical antipsychotics on prolactin elevation are explained by their differential blood-brain disposition: a pharmacological analysis in rats. J Pharm Exp Therapeut 2002;302:1129–1134.
49 Turrone P, Kapur S, Seeman MV, Flint AJ: Elevation of prolactin levels by atypical antipsychotics. Am J Psych 2002;159:133–135.
50 Kapur S, Zipursky R, Jones C, Remington G, Houle S: Relationship between dopamine D2 occupancy, clinical response, and side effects: a double-blind PET study of first episode schizophrenia. Am J Psych 2000;157:514–520.
51 Kapur S, Zipursky R, Jones C, Shammi CS, Remington G, Seeman P: A positron emission tomography study of quetiapine in schizophrenia: a preliminary finding of an antipsychotic effect with only transiently high dopamine D2 receptor occupancy. Arch Gen Psych 2000;57:553–559.
52 Jones C, Kapur S, Remington G, Zipursky R: Transient dopamine d2 occupancy in low EPS-incidence drugs: PET evidence. Biol Psych 2000; 47(suppl):S112.
53 Bushe C, Shaw M, Peveler RC: A review of the association between antipsychotic use and hyperprolactinaemia. J Psychopharmacol 2008;22(suppl):46–55.
54 Paparrigopoulos T, Liappas J, Tzavellas E, Mourikis I, Soldatos C: Amisulpride-induced hyperprolactinaemia is reversible following discontinuation. Prog Neuro-Psychopharmacol Biol Psychiatry 2007;31:92–96.
55 Chue P, Eerdekens M, Augustyns I, Lachaux B, Molcan P, Eriksson I, Pretorius H, David AS: Comparative efficacy and safety of long-acting risperidone and risperidone oral tablets. Eur Neuropsychopharmacol 2005;15:111–117.
56 Lee BH, Kin YK: The relationship between prolactin response and clinical efficacy of risperidone in acute psychotic inpatients. Prog Neuropsychopharmacol Biol Psychiatry 2006;30:658–662.
57 Kinon BJ, Gilmore J, Liu H, Halbreich UM: Prevalence of hyperprolactinaemia in schizophrenic patients treated with conventional antipsychotic medications or risperidone. Psychoneuroendocrinology 2003;28:55–68.

Timothy G. Dinan, MD, PhD, DSc, MRCPsych
Department of Psychiatry
Cork University Hospital, Wilton
Cork (Ireland)
Tel. +353 21 492 2593, Fax +353 21 492 2584 E-Mail t.dinan@ucc.ie

Thakore J, Leonard BE (eds): Metabolic Effects of Psychotropic Drugs.
Mod Trends Pharmacopsychiatry. Basel, Karger, 2009, vol 26, pp 116–128

Impact of Hyperprolactinaemia on the General Health of Patients with Schizophrenia

Hiram J. Wildgust[a] · Dora Kohen[b]

[a]Hiram Consulting, Ackworth, and [b]Lancashire Postgraduate School of Medicine, Preston, UK

Abstract

This paper examines in detail the impact of antipsychotic medication on hyperprolactinaemia and in turn its effect on the physical health of patients treated for schizophrenia. The methodology was a critical review of the published literature, identifying systematic reviews, meta-analyses, population studies, post-marketing surveillance studies, randomized controlled trials (RCTs), observational data and clinical guidelines. The results show that the quality of prolactin data reported in most clinical studies is limited. Hyperprolactinaemia is common in clinical practice. There are emerging concerns relating to secondary hypogonadism and associated consequences of osteoporosis and sexual function. Population studies are now linking raised prolactin with increased risk of hip fractures and possibly breast cancer. In conclusion, hyperprolactinaemia should be considered in the risk balance equation when prescribing antipsychotics. All patients prescribed antipsychotics should be monitored for prolactin levels. It will be important to share this knowledge with health care professionals to ensure that they recognise the symptoms and inform patients, families and carers of the risks. High-quality studies are required to disentangle the risk of fractures and breast cancer from lifestyle, illness factors and treatment effects.

Prolactin (PRL), a hormone secreted by the anterior pituitary, has a major role in regulation processes [1]. It was discovered in 1933 by Riddle et al. [2] in the crops of pigeons and was named as such for its role in lactation. The discovery was not translated into human physiology or clinical understanding until the 1970s and that is when the concept of prolactinaemia arose. Hyperprolactinaemia (HPRL) can be defined simply as sustained levels of PRL higher than normal values. Commonly, HPRL is defined as blood PRL levels of >20 ng/ml for males and >25 ng/ml for females [3].

It is now known that HPRL is the commonest disorder of the hypothalamic-pituitary axis and could be caused by physiological processes as well as pharmacological agents. Furthermore, it has been established that HPRL is associated with side effects such as galactorrhoea, gynaecomastia, hypogonadism and fertility problems, including sexual dysfunction both in men and women [4, 5]. Chronic hypogonadism has been associated with an increased risk of osteoporosis in both sexes, and a possibly increased risk of cardiovascular disorders in young women. Additionally, there are emerging concerns about a possible association of HPRL with breast cancer and pituitary tumours [6, 7].

The focus of this chapter will be to examine in detail the impact of antipsychotic medication on HPRL and in turn its effects on the physical health of patients treated for schizophrenia.

Prolactin Physiology, Regulation and Secretion

PRL a hormone in the regulation of lactation, named by Riddle et al. [2], is today known to have over 300 separate biological activities [1] including reproduction (lactation, leuteal function, reproductive behaviour) and homeostasis (immune response, osmoregulation, angiogenesis). Human PRL consists of 199 amino acids and has similar structure, binding and functional properties as growth hormone [1]. PRL synthesis and secretion in humans is mainly from lactotrope cells in the anterior pituitary gland and is largely regulated by dopamine (inhibitory), although thyrotropin-releasing hormone (PRL release) plays a small role. To a much lesser extent, PRL can be synthesised in several other locations such as the hypothalamus, placenta and mammary gland. The links between the hypothalamus and pituitary gland are important for normal PRL secretion [8] and interference with this linkage will break the inhibitory effect of dopamine resulting in HPRL.

Common Causes of Hyperprolactinaemia

Antipsychotic-associated HPRL is believed to be the commonest cause of raised PRL. However, it is also known that some physiological, pharmacological and pathological mechanisms may also increase PRL.

The main physiological causes of HPRL include pregnancy, acute stress and nipple suckling [9]. Pregnancy in schizophrenia is the most likely reason for HPRL (PRL up to 240 ng/ml) and so needs to be excluded in women presenting with clinical features of HPRL.

A number of drugs other than antipsychotics affect the dopamine system, and as expected are associated with HPRL including anti-emetics, some antidepressants and some analgesics [9]. Electroconvulsive therapy has also been associated with transient PRL elevation [10]. In many centres retrospective diagnosis of possible epileptic seizure is done by measuring the post-ictal PRL levels.

One of the rare but important causes of HPRL is prolactinoma which usually presents with elevated PRL levels of >100 ng/ml (2,100 IU/l) [11].

Holt [9] raises the hypothesis that dysregulation of dopamine control of PRL secretion may be an important aetiological factor in the development of prolactinomas.

Other disease states associated with HPRL include primary hypothyroidism, chest wall lesions, chronic renal failure, cirrhosis of the liver, ectopic secretion of PRL, seizures and cancer metastases [12].

The Impact of Antipsychotics on Prolactin Elevation

Antipsychotic blockade of D2 receptors on the anterior pituitary lactotrope is the main mechanism by which antipsychotics increase PRL. Kapur and Seeman [13] suggested that fast dissociation from the D_2 receptor makes an antipsychotic more accommodating of physiological dopamine transmission, permitting an antipsychotic effect without PRL elevation. Seeman [14] showed that the blockade of D2 receptors by typical antipsychotics is more prolonged than with atypicals and this leads to the accumulation of PRL.

Kapur et al. [15] hypothesised that atypical antipsychotics with a propensity for PRL elevation would show a higher pituitary versus striatal D2 receptor occupancy and in part would reflect their ease at crossing the blood-brain barrier. Additionally, it is now recognised that some of the metabolites of antipsychotics themselves may have an effect on PRL elevation such as the 9-hydroxy metabolite of risperidone which has a predominant role in PRL elevation.

The work of Green et al. [16] and Kuruvilla et al. [17] support the view that schizophrenia is not associated with raised PRL elevation in unmedicated patients. PRL elevation starts with antipsychotic treatment. Research to date shows that all antipsychotics have been associated with varying degrees of HPRL [18]; however, it is still important to note that antipsychotics show differences in terms of rates, severity and sustained levels of raised PRL [4, 18].

The quality of PRL data reported in many clinical trials is limited [19]. Few trials have PRL as a primary outcome measure, categorical levels are rarely reported, and few studies report both PRL and gonadal hormones. Most studies fail to monitor blood levels for antipsychotics and hence where a decline in PRL is reported over time, it is difficult to tease out if this is a real effect or just a reflection of non- compliance. Bushe et al. [19] identified those studies reporting categorical rates of HPRL showing a range of 42–92% in females and 18–72% in males. This confirms that HPRL is a common side effect of antipsychotic medication with females being more prone. Byerly et al. [4] suggested a clinically valuable categorisation of antipsychotics into two groups: those associated with marked and sustained PRL elevation (some typical and some atypical antipsychotic) and those second-generation antipsychotics which appear to have little effect on PRL levels.

There has been a long-held view that typical antipsychotics are associated with markedly high rates of HPRL; however, an examination of the literature questions this view. Bushe and Shaw [20] found that in clinical practice the rates of HPRL in male and female patients on monotherapy with typical antipsychotics were only 33%.

Similar rates for HPRL are shown in several other studies [21, 22] thus illustrating that many patients on typical antipsychotics do not show HPRL. The rates of HPRL reported by Bushe et al. [19] were considerably lower for typicals than for the atypicals amisulpride and risperidone.

There are a number of studies which have examined the long-term impact of antipsychotics on PRL levels. Meltzer and Fang [23] reported that within 72 h men and women on phenothiazines, would show 3.2- and 3.8-fold increases in PRL levels, respectively, and these would remain elevated at 1 and 3 months during the observation period. Within 48–96 h of stopping the medication PRL levels would normalise. Chouinard et al. [24] reported that there was no evidence of growing tolerance to PRL-elevating antipsychotics in those patients who had been treated for many years with these medications. In contrast, Brown and Laughren [25] reported tolerance after 4 months of treatment with typicals. The discrepancy in these findings may be associated with issues of compliance rather than tolerance.

Svestka et al. [26] reported one of the few studies with atypical antipsychotics where PRL was the primary outcome measure. Amisulpride and risperidone PRL levels increased significantly in 100% of female patients as early as the first week of treatment, whereas with quetiapine and zotepine, PRL levels were reduced as early as the first week after treatment. In the same study, olanzapine was associated with mild transient PRL elevation. In this study, PRL elevation did not correlate with age, menopausal status, efficacy of the antipsychotic, daily dose, serum lipids or blood glucose levels.

Clinical Adverse Effects of Prolactin

Halbreich and Kahn [3] proposed that many of the clinical adverse consequences of HPRL could be accounted for by its effects on the HPG axis. HPRL is associated with suppression of gonadotropin pulsatile release, which in turn inhibits the release of luteinizing hormone (LH) and follicle-stimulating hormone (FSH) from the pituitary leading to suppression of ovarian and testicular function in turn leading to hypogonadism [3, 27]. This potentially further led to a range of menstrual disorders, reduced fertility in both sexes, decreased sexual function in men and women including decreased libido, increased risk of cardiovascular disorders, galactorrhoea, anxiety and depression. Halbreich and Kahn [3] also postulated that adverse events such as an increased risk of breast cancer were possibly associated with HPRL. This hypothesis is supported by Harvey et al. [6] who identified that PRL has a direct action on breast tissue where it can act as a mitogen in the mammary gland. Furthermore, PRL stimulates the growth and motility of human breast cancer and acts as a potent survival factor protecting human breast cancer cells from apoptosis.

The last decade has seen a new research focus on the secondary impact of antipsychotics on gonadal hormones and hypogonadism through HPRL in schizophrenia. Smith et al. [22] reported the impact of typical antipsychotics, with a 2-year minimum exposure on patients with schizophrenia, finding that 75% of the females and 34% of the males have HPRL. The rates of hypogonadism were 85% and 6.4% in females and males, respectively. This highlights that PRL levels are a relatively good indicator of risk of hypogonadism, but in females suggests that HPRL levels at the top end of the normal range may also indicate hypogonadism. Howes et al. [28] investigated 103 patients with schizophrenia or schizoaffective disorder with a medium treatment duration of 3.3 years with antipsychotics. The rates of hypogonadism in females was 79%, and 92% of the women had hypo-oestrogenism and 28% of the men showed hypotestosteronism.

Common Side-Effects Associated with Antipsychotic-Induced Hyperprolactinaemia

Gynaecomastia and Galactorrhoea

It is important to note that there are no standardised methods for measuring galactorrhoea. Beumont et al. [29] describe massaging the breast for 3 min and then measuring the volume of milk produced. Others use a milk pump to extract milk and or just simply ask the patient. Prior to the introduction of antipsychotic medication in the 1950s neither galactorrhoea nor gynaecomastia had been noted as important complaints from patients with schizophrenia. However, Robinson [30] found an incidence rate for galactorrhoea of 10%, while Plante and Roy [31] reported an incidence rate of 57%. Tolis et al. [32] reported 65 cases of galactorrhoea and found that there was no correlation between PRL levels and the frequency and severity of galactorrhoea. Beumont et al. [29] pointed out that the correlation between raised PRL and lactation is not a direct one as other factors were involved in the initiation and maintenance of galactorrhoea.

More recent studies suggest that the incidence of galactorrhoea in clinical practice is lower than earlier reports. Wesselmann and Windgassen [33] completed one of the first prospective studies of galactorrhoea in schizophrenia in 150 patients. They reported that an incidence rate of 14% and prevalence rate of 19% and galactorrhoea occurred between the 7th and 75th days after initiating treatment. Only 28% of their patients spontaneously disclosed these side effects to their psychiatrists as they found this embarrassing. Underreporting and under recognition of symptoms could be one of the underlying factors in the great variety of reported prevalence and incidence of this adverse effect. Wesselmann and Windgassen [33] stated that more than half of his female patients who experienced galactorrhoea closely linked this to their femininity. They had 1 patient who misinterpreted this as pseudo-pregnancy. Galactorrhoea is reported much less commonly in males with rates around 1%. However, Halbreich and Kahn [3] reported that up to 33% of men with HPRL actually had galactorrhoea on examination. It is clear that galactorrhoea should not be left to self-reporting and be included in the physical examination of the patient.

Menstrual Cycle and Fertility

Menstrual dysfunction associated with psychoses was recognised well before the introduction of antipsychotics [34]. These early observations supported the view that illness and possibly life style factors also played a role in menstrual abnormalities, separate from the effects of antipsychotics on low oestrogen via hypogonadism. The rates of amenorrhoea vary widely between studies, ranging from very low figures to as high 78% as reported by Smith et al. [22], and averaging around the 30% level. This wide variation in rates may be a consequence of the definition of amenorrhoea. It has been defined as the temporary or permanent absence of menstruation for more than 6 months. Wong and Seeman [35] defined amenorrhoea as 3 consecutive missed periods. Hence, many pharmacological studies in schizophrenia designed for 12 weeks or less would miss clinical signs of adverse events of the menstrual cycle. Wong and Seeman [35] highlighted that 90% of the women linked normal menstruation with good health and subjects with irregular menses had significantly lower self-esteem than those with normal menses ($p < 0.01$). In the same study, patients with amenorrhoea had higher PRL levels than those without (57 vs. 27 ng/ml).

Smith et al. [22] followed up patients who had been stabilised on typical antipsychotics for at least 2 years measuring both PRL levels as well as gonadal hormones. Although the average dose of antipsychotics in chlorpromazine equivalents was only 384 mg, 75% of the females had PRL levels greater than the upper limit of normal, 36% had amenorrhoea, 32% oligomenorrhoea and 36% had apparent normal menstruation; however, only 37% of these women were actually ovulating. Furthermore, this study showed that HPRL in women was correlated with the degree of suppression of the HPG axis. Howes et al. [28] found similarly high levels of intermittent anovulatory cycles (92%) in a population of premenopausal females with a median exposure to antipsychotic of 3.3 years.

In clinical practice, menstrual disturbance is the most obvious feature of HPRL and has been traditionally used as a clinical sign for raised PRL. Smith et al. [22] and Howes et al. [28] demonstrated that many women with apparently regular menstruation would not be ovulating, indicating a hypogonadal state.

With the appearance of antipsychotics with a lower propensity for raised PRL levels and amenorrhoea, clinicians should also recognise that switching to these medications may initiate ovulation and put the patient at risk of unplanned pregnancy.

Osteoporosis is defined by the WHO as at least a fall of 2.5 SDs below the mean peak bone density for young adults and osteopenia is defined as bone density between <2.5 and >1.0 SD.

Prior to the introduction of antipsychotics, there were not many reports of fractures or osteopenia/osteoporosis in patients with schizophrenia, except for a few case reports of hip fractures in patients undergoing unmodified electroconvulsive therapy.

A great deal of our current knowledge and understanding about the risks of developing osteopenia/osteoporosis or fractures associated with HPRL comes from animal studies and reports of patients with pituitary tumours.

Little is known about the putative role of PRL on bone cells and bone formation in humans [36]. Adler et al. [37] investigated the effects of PRL excess and estrogen deficiency on bone in rats and concluded that HPRL with osteoporosis is likely to be due to PRL-induced hypogonadism rather than a direct effect of PRL on calcium homeostasis. Amenorrhoea associated with HPRL was the first recognised model of functional hypogonadal osteoporosis [38] showing an association with decrease cortical and trabecular bone density. Other recognised associations are smoking, lack of exercise and lithium-induced hyperparathyroidism [39]. Klibanski et al. [38] were the first to highlight that young women were vulnerable to developing osteopenia/osteoporosis. There are several studies of patients diagnosed with pituitary tumours who report increased rates of bone loss. Biller et al. [40] found that bone density decreased significantly in HPRL women who were amenorrheic for more than 20 months. This suggests that studies in treatment pathways in schizophrenia should continue for at least 2 years to pick up these phenomena. Further, it does confirm the clinical importance of amenorrhoea as a risk factor for osteoporosis and osteopenia. Greenspan et al. [41] confirmed that osteoporosis developed in men with hyperprolactinaemic hypogonadism.

O'Keane [27] points out that prior to 2000, there were no studies in schizophrenia which examined the relationship between hypogonadism, secondary to HPRL and bone density. The clinical trials in this area have been well described and reviewed by several authors including Leucht et al. [42] and Byerly et al. [4]. Overall, there is a consistency of findings amongst these reviewers. Albeit limited by small cohorts and short duration, these studies show that patients with schizophrenia, on antipsychotics over a prolonged period of time, report increased rates of osteoporosis and osteopenia.

Kishimoto et al. [43] reports a study in 74 male patients (mean age 58.9) with schizophrenia, investigating the possible causes of reduced bone mineral density. They report that 37% had osteopenia and 27% osteoporosis, 87% of the subjects had HPRL and vitamin D levels were normal. Exercise and vitamin D did not protect these patients from lower bone mineral density. The high PRL group showed low levels of FSH and LH, and significantly low gonadal hormones. The results of this study support the hypothesis that HPRL impacts on the HPG axis which contributes to bone loss and the greatest bone loss correlated with the increased duration of HPRL. Vekemans and Robyn [44] highlighted that in men PRL levels rise with age, whereas in women PRL levels decline with age and by the time men are 60, their normal PRL levels are higher than women of similar ages. This observation raises the important question of increased risks in older men.

Howard et al. [45] completed the first large- scale population study to investigate patients with a history of schizophrenia and risk of hip fracture. The method used was a case-controlled study comparing hip fractures in the general practice research database (n = 16,341) with matched controls (n = 29,889). The key finding was that hip fractures were significantly associated with a diagnosis of schizophrenia (OR 1.73; 95% CI 1.32–2.28) and independently associated with PRL elevating antipsychotics (OR = 2.6; 95% CI 2.43–2.78). This is one of the main studies to show that schizophrenia has to be recognized as a significant risk factor for hip fractures.

Breast Cancer

Leucht et al. [42], in a systematic review of physical illness in schizophrenia, found that population studies which examined the relationship between schizophrenia and breast cancer were inconclusive. They also examined the question of whether high PRL levels promote breast cancer. Their findings supported the view that the evidence for this was discordant. This chapter explores new findings which were not included in the review by Leucht et al. [42].

Catts et al. [46] completed one of the first meta-analysis of cancer incidence rates in schizophrenia which included 100,000 patients and 70,000 parents and 73,000 siblings. This meta-analysis showed that the incidence of breast cancer was significantly increased in female patients SIR = 1.12 (CI 1.02–1.23; p = 0.02). In parents of patients with schizophrenia or their siblings, the pooled data for all cancers were shown to be significantly reduced in parents: SIR = 0.90 (CI 0.88–0.93) and siblings SIR = 0.89 (CI 0.84–0.94). These findings are consistent with genes associated with schizophrenia, being protective against cancers.

Hippisley-Cox et al. [47] report an epidemiological study using the QRESEARCH database (UK primary care clinical records). The population consisted of roughly 4 million patients with nearly 18.7 million person year's observation. The study showed an increased risk of breast cancer in patients with schizophrenia (adjusted OR 1.52 for deprivation, smoking, obesity and use of other medications, 95% CI 1.10–2.11).

This study differs from many of the earlier studies as it included many patients aged >50 years. Since breast cancer is more common in older women, it is likely that a greater powered study would be required to detect increased rates of breast cancer in younger women.

Hankinson et al. [48] investigated the risk of breast cancer associated with high PRL by doing a series of epidemiological studies now well known as the US Nurse Health Study. This study cohort was establishes in 1976 with 121,700 US female registered nurses (30–55 years) and followed up every 2 years. From 1989 through 1990 blood samples for different blood biochemistry including PRL results were collected from 32.826 women. Hankinson et al. [48] observed a significant association with observed PRL levels and postmenopausal breast cancer (highest versus lowest quartile multivariate relative risk of 2.02; 95% CI 1.24–3.31). Hankinson along with Tworoger have now published a series of papers which show increase risk of breast cancer both in premenopausal and postmenopausal women. This is probably the strongest clinical evidence supporting the view that elevated PRL is a risk factor for breast cancer.

Harvey et al. [6] believe that the balance of evidence from in vitro and animal studies now supports the view that raised PRL is associated with breast cancer. Furthermore, they challenge the long-held view that findings from animal data may not be applicable to humans. These findings are now being included in some of the summary of product characteristics in the US for some of the antipsychotics. There are some confounds with the PRL story, as there is laboratory evidence that trifluoperazine inhibits the development of cancer cells.

Halbreich et al. [49] identified high rates of breast cancer in patients with chronic schizophrenia who were screened with mammography. Wernicke et al. [50] completed one of the first studies to assess breast screening for patients with schizophrenia. Overall, they found psychiatric patients with a diagnosis of psychosis (OR = 0.33, CI 0.18–0.61; $p < 0.01$) were less like to attend for breast screening than the general population.

Both studies highlight the importance of breast screening in patients with schizophrenia.

In conclusion, findings from a meta-analysis suggests that schizophrenia maybe protective of breast cancer in parents and siblings, but breast cancer rates were significantly increased in female patients. Epidemiological studies by Hankinson and Tworoger provide strong evidence supporting the thesis that higher levels of PRL potentially put patients at increased risk of breast cancer.

Hyperprolactinaemia and Sexual Dysfunction

Sexual dysfunction is associated with a wide variety of possible mechanisms. Gitlin [51] described the possible effects of a direct CNS effect on the neurotransmitter system, sedation secondary to histamine, a peripheral effect resulting in priaprism, and hormonal effects primarily through HPRL.

In patients with schizophrenia, it is extremely difficult to disentangle the sexual dysfunction caused by HPRL from the psychopathology of schizophrenia and the impact of antipsychotics and other medication on a variety of receptor systems such as serotonin and histamine. Weizman et al. [52] conducted a study to look at sexual dysfunction associated with HPRL patients with renal failure undergoing haemodialysis. They noted that patients with high levels of PRL (130 ng/ml) as compared to patients with low levels of PRL (36.3 ng/ml) were clinically impotent. On treatment with bromocriptine, 4 males and 1 female showed a restoration of sexual desire and potency. These findings support the hypothesis that HPRL can be a major cause for reversible sexual dysfunction. Smith et al. [53] published one of the first controlled studies investigating the frequency and underlying mechanisms of sexual dysfunction in people on antipsychotics. Sexual dysfunction occurred in 45% of patients taking antipsychotics and 17% of non-treated controls. They concluded that HPRL was the main cause of sexual dysfunction in females (with 75% of the women being HPRL) whereas in males (with 34% of the men being HPRL) autonomic side effects were a dominant cause of sexual dysfunction but in those men with HPRL this superseded other causes of sexual dysfunction.

Howes et al. [28] investigated the relationship between sexual function and gonadal hormones. Although this study showed high rates of sexual dysfunction and high rates of hypogonadism (92% women and 28% men) there was no correlation between sexual function and gonadal hormones which indicated that this is not the main aetiological factor in these cases. Costa et al. [54] reported no differences in sexual function between patients treated with the atypical antipsychotic olanzapine and conventional antipsychotics but they did show differences in the rate of normalisation of hormone levels. This illustrates that sexual function is a complex multi-factorial activity controlled by many different neurotransmitters and not just PRL.

Clinical Management of Hyperprolactinaemia

Historically, it was considered that a raised PRL in association with typical antipsychotics was almost inevitable. This gave rise to a nihilistic perspective, which ignored HPRL in patients unless they complained of adverse events. With the advent of newer antipsychotics with a lower risk of HPRL this perspective is no longer valid.

It is now recognised that raised PRL is not benign and the risk of HPRL can be reduced through screening and planned antipsychotic treatments.

HPRL and its clinical side effects have not received all the attention they deserve. The symptoms and sexual side effects of HPRL have not been fully clinically recognized or sufficiently investigated. There are still male and female patients who are not checked for their PRL levels, who do not complain to their GPs or the community key workers in the mental health teams and who suffer silently.

The first step in recognition of the symptoms and side effects in the community will be the training of GPs and non-medical professionals in primary care trusts in gathering the information and recognizing the side effects in patients who may be unwilling to discuss the issues or who may not be aware of the impact of the medication.

Community mental health nurses, key workers and community pharmacist should be involved in assessing the problem.

The next step should be to measure PRL levels routinely, on initiating antipsychotic treatment and during the stabilisation period as part of patients physical health screen. This should be followed by training in recognition and follow-up of the longer-term systemic and metabolic side effects of the medication including establishment of osteoporosis and breast problems as early as possible.

For all these the patients, their families and carers should be involved in understanding the side effects and in asking the relevant questions.

Medical management and psychiatrists should make the case for financial resources when necessary. There are several guidelines on the monitoring and management of PRL in schizophrenia, but few offer practical advice [55]. Peveler et al. [56] put together some clinical recommendations on antipsychotic-associated HPRL based on a critical appraisal of the current literature. Their main recommendation was that PRL elevation appeared to be of greatest concern in people under the age of 25 years as they are at greatest risk of subsequent osteoporosis. HPRL should be avoided in those with a history of breast cancer, possibly prostate cancer, prolactinomas and those diagnosed with osteoporosis. HPRL should also be avoided in women planning pregnancy. Clinicians should consider giving patients information about the risks of elevated PRL, particularly osteoporosis, reduced fertility, menstrual irregularities and sexual dysfunction.

Peveler et al. [56] suggest that in any patients presenting with PRL levels greater than 150 ng/ml, a prolactinoma should be considered and the patients should be referred to a specialist endocrinologist.

Hopefully, the data of PRL will now been translated from basic sciences to clinical practice and will lead to better quality of life and life expectancy for patients at risk of developing HPRL.

References

1 Freeman ME, Kanyicska B, Lerant A, Nagy G: Prolactin: structure, function, and regulation of secretion. Physiol Rev 2000;80:1523–1631.

2 Riddle O, Bates RW, Dykshorn SW: The preparation, identification and assay of prolactin: a hormone of the anterior pituitary. Am J Physiol 1933; 105:191–216.

3 Halbreich U, Kahn LS: Hyperprolactinemia and schizophrenia: mechanisms and clinical aspects. J Psychiatr Pract 2003;9:344–353.

4 Byerly M, Suppes T, Tran Q, Baker RA: Clinical implications of antipsychotic-induced hyperprolactinaemia in Patients with schizophrenia and bipolar spectrum disorder. J Clin Psychiatry 2007;27:639–661.

5 Haddad PM, Wieck A: Antipsychotic-induced hyperprolactinaemia mechanisms, clinical features and management. Drugs 2004;64:2291–2314.

6 Harvey PW, Everett DJ, Springall CJ: Adverse effects of prolactin in rodents and humans: breast and prostate cancer. J Psychopharmacol 2008;22:20–27.

7 Szarfman A, Tonning JM, Levine JG, Doraiswamy PM: Atypical antipsychotics and pituitary tumours: a pharmacovigilance study. Pharmacotherapy 2006; 26:748–758.

8 Ben-Jonathan N, Hnasko R: Dopamine as a prolactin (PRL) inhibitor. Endocr Rev 2001;22:724–763.

9 Holt RIG: Medical causes and consequences of hyperprolactinaemia. J Psychopharmacol 2008;22: 28–37.

10 Pritchard PB 3rd, Wannamaker BB, Sagel J, Nair R, Devillier C: Endocrine function following complex partial seizures. Ann Neurol 1983;14:27–32.
11 Serri O, Chik CL, Ur E, Ezzat S: Diagnosis and management of hyperprolactinemia. CMAJ 2003;169:575–581.
12 Liu JK, Couldwell WT: Contemporary management of prolactinomas. Neurosurg Focus 2004;16:1–11.
13 Kapur S, Seeman P: Does fast dissociation from the D2 recptor explain the action of atypical antipsychotics? A New Hypothesis. Am J Psychiatry 2001;158:360–369.
14 Seeman P: Atypical antipsychotics: mechanism of action. Focus, 2004. Am Psychiatr Assoc 2004;2:48–58.
15 Kapur S, Langlois X, Vinken P, Megens AAHP, De Coster R, Andrews JS: The differential effects of atypical antipsychotics on prolactin elevation are explained by their differential blood-brain disposition: a pharmacological analysis in rats. J Pharmacol Exp Ther 2002;302:1129–1134.
16 Green AI, Faraone SV, Brown WA: Prolactin shifts after neuroleptic withdrawal. Psychiatr Res 1990;32:213–219.
17 Kuruvilla A, Peedicayil J, Srikrishna G, Kuruvilla K, Kanagasabapathy AS: A study of serum prolactin levels in schizophrenia: comparison of males and females. Clin Exp Pharmacol Physiol 1992;19:603–606.
18 Turrone P, Kapur S, Seeman MV, Flint AJ: Elevation of prolactin levels by atypical antipsychotics. Am J Psychiatry 2002;159:133–135.
19 Bushe C, Shaw M, Peveler R: A review of the association between antipsychotics and hyperprolactinaemia. J Psychopharmacol 2008;22:46–55.
20 Bushe C, Shaw M: Prevalence of hyperprolactinaemia in a naturalistic cohort of schizophrenia and bipolar outpatients during treatment with typical and atypical antipsychotics. J Psychopharmacol 2007;21:768–773.
21 Kinon BJ, Gilmore JA, Liu H, Halbreich UM:. Prevalence of hyperprolactinemia in schizophrenic patients treated with conventional antipsychotic medications or risperidone. Psychoneuroendocrinology 2003;28(suppl 2):55–68.
22 Smith S, Wheeler MJ, Murray R, O'Keane V: The effects of antipsychotic-induced hyperprolactinaemia on hypothalamic-pituitary-gonadal-axis. J Clin Psychopharmacol 2002;22:109–114.
23 Meltzer HY, Fang VS: The effect of neuroleptics on serum prolactin in schizophrenic patients. Arch Gen Psychiatry 1976;33:279–286.
24 Chouinard G, Annable L, Jones BD, Collu R: Lack of tolerance to long-term neuroleptic treatment in dopamine tuberoinfundibular system. Acta Psychiatr Scand 1981;64:353–362.
25 Brown WA, Laughren TP: Tolerance to the prolactin-elevating effect of neuroleptics. Psychiatry Res 1981;5:317–322.
26 Svestka J, Synek O, Tomanová J, Rodáková I, Cejpková A: Differences in the effect of second-generation antipsychotics on prolactinaemia: six weeks open-label trial in female in-patients. Neuro Endocrinol Lett 2007;28:381–888.
27 O'Keane V: Antipsychotic-induced hyperprolactinaemia, hypogonadism and osteoporosis in the treatment of schizophrenia. J Psychopharmacol 2008;22:70–75.
28 Howes OD, Wheeler MJ, Pilowsky LS, Landa S, Murray RM, Smith S: Sexual function and gonadal hormones in patients taking antipsychotic treatment for schizophrenia or schizoaffective disorder. J Clin Psychiatry 2007;3:361–367.
29 Beumont PJ, Gelder MG, Friesen HG, Harris G, Mackinnon P, Mandelbrote BM, Wiles JM: The effects of phenothiazines on endocrine function: I. Patients with inappropriate lactation and amenorrhoea. Br J Psychiatry 1974;124:413–419.
30 Robinson B: Breast changes in the male and female with chlorpromazine or reserpine therapy. Med J Aust 1957;44:239–241.
31 Plante N, Roy P: Galactorrhea and neuroleptics. Laval Med 1967;38:103–107.
32 Tolis G, Somma M, Van Campenhout J, Friesen H: Prolactin secretion in sixty-five patients with galactorrhea. Am J Obstet Gynecol 1974;118:91–101.
33 Wesselmann U, Windgassen K: Galactorrhea: subjective response by schizophrenic patients. Acta Psychiatr Scand 1995;91:152–155.
34 Kohen D, Wildgust HJ: Evolution of hyperprolactinaemia as an entity. J Psychopharmacol 2008;22:6–11.
35 Wong J, Seeman MV: Prolactin, menstrual irregularities, quality of life. Schizophr Res 2007;91:270–271.
36 Clément-Lacroix P, Ormandy C, Lepescheux L, Ammann P, Damotte D, Goffin V, Bouchard B, Amling M, Gaillard-Kelly M, Binart N, Baron N, Kelly PA: Osteoblasts are a new target for prolactin: analysis of bone formation in prolactin receptor knockout mice. Endocrinology 1999;140:96–105.
37 Adler RA, Evani R, Mansouri A, Krieg RJ Jr: Relative effects of prolactin excess and estrogen deficiency on bone in rats. Metabolism 1998;47:425–428.
38 Klibanski A, Neer RM, Beitins IZ, Ridgeway EC, Zervas NT, McArthur JW: Decreased bone density in hyperprolactinemic women. N Engl J Med 1980;303:1511–1514.
39 Misra M, Papakostas GI, Kliabanski A: Effects of psychiatric disorders and psychotropic medication on prolactin and bone metabolism. J Clin Psychiatry 2004;65:1607–1618.

40 Biller BM, Baum HB, Rosenthal DI, Saxe VC, Charpie PM, Klibanski A: Progressive trabecular osteopenia in women with hyperprolactinemic amenorrhea. J Clin Endocrinol Metab 1992;75:692–697.
41 Greenspan SL, Neer RM, Ridgway EC, Klibanski A: Osteoporosis in men with hyperprolactinemic hypogonadism. Ann Intern Med 1986;104:777–782.
42 Leucht S, Burkard T, Henderson JH, Maj M, Sartorius N: Physical Illness and Schizophrenia. London, Cambridge Press, 2007.
43 Kishimoto T, Watanabe K, Shimado N, Makita K, Yagi G, Kashima H: Antipsychotic-induced hyperprolactinemia inhibits the hypothalamo-pituitary-gonadal axis and reduces bone mineral density in males patients with schizophrenia. J Clin Psychiatry 2008;69:385–391.
44 Vekemans M, Robyn C: Influence of age on serum prolactin levels in women and men. Br Med J 1975;iv:738–739.
45 Howard L, Kirkwood G, Leese M: Risk of hip fracture in patients with a history of schizophrenia. Br J Psychiatry 2007;190:129–134.
46 Catts VS, Catts SV, O'Toole BI, Frost AD: Cancer incidence in patients with schizophrenia and their first degree relatives: meta-analysis. Acta Psychiatr Scand 2008;117:323–336.
47 Hippisley-Cox J, Vinogradova Y, Coupland C, Parker C: Risk of malignancy in patients with schizophrenia or bipolar disorder. Arch Psychiatry 2007;60:1368–1376.
48 Hankinson SE, Willett WC, Michaud DS, Manson JE, Coldit GA, Longcope C, Rosne B, Speize FE: Plasma prolactin levels and subsequent risk of breast cancer in postmenopausal women. J Natl Cancer Inst 1999;91:629–634.
49 Halbreich U, Shen J, Panaro V: Are chronic psychiatric patients at increased risk for developing breast cancer? Am J Psychiatry 1996;153:559–560.
50 Werneke U, Horn O, Maryon-Davis A, Wessely S, Donnan S, McPherson K: Uptake of screening for breast cancer in patients with mental health problems. J Epidemiol Community Health 2006;60:600–605.
51 Gitlin MJ: Psychotropic medications and their effects on sexual function: diagnosis, biology and treatment approaches. J Clin Psychiatry 1994;55:406–413.
52 Weizman R, Weizman A, Levi J, Gura V, Zevin D, Maoz B, Wijsenbeek H, Ben David M: Sexual dysfunction associated with hyperprolactinemia in males and females undergoing hemodialysis. Psychosom Med 1983;45:259–269.
53 Smith S, O'Keane V, Murray R: Sexual dysfunction in patients taking conventional antipsychotic medication. Br J Psychiatry 2002;181:49–55.
54 Costa AMN, Silvia de Lima M, Filjp SR, Reis de Olivera I, Jesus Mari J: A naturalistic, 9 month follow-up, comparing olanzapine and conventional antipsychotics in sexual function and hormonal profile of males with schizophrenia. J Psychopharmacol 2006;20:6–19.
55 Citrome L: Current guidelines and their recommendations for prolactin monitoring in psychosis. J Psychopharmacol 2008;22:90–97.
56 Peveler RC, Branford D, Citrome L, Fitzgerald P, Harvey PW, Holt RIG, Howard L, Jones I, Kohen D, O'Keane V, Pariante C, Pendlebury J, Smith S, Yeomans D: Antipsychotic associated hyperprolactinaemia: clinical recommendations. J Psychopharmacol 2008;22:98–103.

Hiram J. Wildgust, PhD
Hiram Consulting
11, Cricketers Close
Ackworth WF7 7PW (UK)
Tel./Fax +44 1977 615 208, E-Mail awildpainter@aol.com

Author Index

Subject Index